SUSTAINABLE HEALTH

SUSTAINABLE HEALTH

Simple Habits to Transform Your Life

Susan L. Roberts

W. W. Norton & Company
Independent Publishers Since 1923
New York • London

Important Note: Sustainable Health is intended to provide general information on the subject of health and well-being; it is not a substitute for medical or psychological treatment and may not be relied upon for purposes of diagnosing or treating any illness. Please seek out the care of a professional healthcare provider if you are pregnant, nursing, or experiencing symptoms of any potentially serious condition.

For information about permission to reproduce selections from this book, write to Permissions, W. W. Norton & Company, Inc., 500 Fifth Avenue, New York, NY 10110

For information about special discounts for bulk purchases, please contact W. W. Norton Special Sales at specialsales@wwnorton.com or 800-233-4830

Manufacturing by LSC Willard
Book design by Molly Heron
Production manager: Katelyn MacKenzie

Library of Congress Cataloging-in-Publication Data

Names: Roberts, Susan L., 1951– author.
Title: Sustainable health : simple habits to transform your life / Susan L. Roberts.
Description: New York : W.W. Norton & Company, 2018. | Includes bibliographical references and index.
Identifiers: LCCN 2018019203 | ISBN 9780393712834 (pbk.)
Subjects: LCSH: Self-care, Health—Popular works. | Nutrition—Popular works. | Mind and body—Popular works.
Classification: LCC RA776.95 .R59 2018 | DDC 613.2—dc23
LC record available at https://lccn.loc.gov/2018019203

W. W. Norton & Company, Inc., 500 Fifth Avenue, New York, N.Y. 10110
www.wwnorton.com

W. W. Norton & Company Ltd., 15 Carlisle Street, London W1D 3BS

1 2 3 4 5 6 7 8 9 0

Contents

Acknowledgments

EACH TIME I write a book I'm reminded of the words Mark Twain wrote for Huckleberry Finn, " . . . if I'd a knowed what a trouble it was to make a book I wouldn't a tackled it . . ." and I remember how often Twain returned to the task again. Fortunately, a lot of people make it possible to tackle writing a book and I would like to thank some of those who helped me.

First, I'd like to thank my editor, Deborah Malmud. Our chance meeting and brief conversation opened the door to an amazing year of research and integration of ideas that transformed thirty years of thoughts about healing into a coherent approach. I am grateful that through her, the legacy of W.W. Norton stands behind me in this endeavor. Kate Prince, who assisted with editing, patiently answered questions and held my hand through a few panicky moments when I wondered if I'd meet my deadline and word count. Mariah Eppes worked with the manuscript throughout Irene Vartanoff's excellent copyediting. Deborah and all the editorial staff helped steer the original book into what I believe will be a much more useful workbook.

Grand Master Nan Lu, OMD, and the staff of the Tao of Healing Center in New York City introduced me to Five Element Theory, which provided an essential key to developing the Healing Compass. Elaine Katen read some early (and ultimately discarded) chapters and shared these with Dr. Lu. I believe the book is much the better for their early critiques. Dr. Lu, Elaine, Irma Jenne, Deborah Hallahan, and Tatiana Phillipova all taught me to look beyond the body and even the mind to the spiritual essence present in all things. I could never have written this book but for them teaching me to appreciate the power of *Qi*. Any errors or liberties I've taken with Five Element Theory rest solely on my shoulders and reflect my limitations, not theirs.

A brief conversation about cultural appropriation that I had with Shannon Shula at the outset of writing made me rethink using "medicine wheels." That birthed the Healing Compass, which became the heart of this book. The book is much stronger because I claim my own cultural heritage.

Frank Rowsome and Nancy Buchenauer read over an early version of the introduction and pointed out some of the finer points of philosophy and physics that kept me on track with the academics of these subjects. Any transgressions in physics or philosophy represent my own limited knowledge, not theirs.

Many friends and family read or listened to various versions of the chapters and gave me important feedback: Esther Bell, Fran Brazzell, Dan Brecher, Elena Camerin Young, Alicia Canary, Michelle Colletti, Holly Coryell, Gwen Goodman, Kristin Graves, Carlos Henninger, Carol Hohman, Tara Krupich, Liz Langone, Kay Mann, Hermine Meinhard, Gabriela Montequin, Roberta Raeburn, Vaness Rolón, Graeme Roberts, Harold Roberts, Leila Saad, Mike Savage, Marsha Stone, Lynn Temenski, and Laurie Treinkman. They all helped me fine tune some points and make the text more understandable.

A number of people volunteered to try out the Sustainable Health program before I got down to writing about it. A special shout out to those intrepid souls whose feedback was so helpful in the beginning stages: Janet Juntunen, Roberta Raeburn, Alicia Canary, Kristin Graves, Brenda Lew, Noelle Everhart, Heather Jackson-Peña, Kay Jamison, Laura Lin, Annette Reid, Robin Coryell, and Marti Capuco.

Over the course of four decades as an occupational therapist, I have had the great good fortune to have had many clients who taught me so much. Likewise, the students I met teaching in university occupational therapy departments also enriched my life and experience. They, too, make up some of the fabric of this book. I hope I have given as much as I got in return.

Dr. Lu often asks his students, "Who stands behind you?" When he does this he refers to our lineage of teachers. I owe a great debt to those teachers who stood behind me as I wrote this book. From Harvard Divinity School: Katie Geneva Cannon taught me to question the source of ethical stances; Karen McCarthy Brown introduced me to Afro-Caribbean healing traditions; Veena Das shed a new light on anthropology by viewing it through a Hindu perspective; Jane Smith taught by example the ways of negotiating a large institution;

Jo Ann Hackett, Michael Coogan, and Peter Lambdin brought the ancient Near East to life in all its similarities and differences; Sheila Briggs illuminated the early centuries of the Modern Era with a powerful feminist perspective; and Clarissa Atkinson did the same for the Middle Ages.

At Boston University's Sargent College, Nancy Talbot introduced me to developmental theory. Cathy Trombly opened the door to the healing powers of occupational therapy, and Whitney Powers shared his delight in the magnificence of human anatomy.

My high school chemistry teacher, Robert George Riddell, in Kents Hill, Maine, instilled a love of science and taught me how to deconstruct equations, something that has been immensely useful during the course of this book. Last but not least, I thank my first grade teacher Ms. English, in Overland Park, Kansas. She taught me to read, and I have used that skill every day of my life since then.

Preface

To raise new questions, new possibilities, to regard old problems from a new angle, requires creative imagination and marks real advance in science.

—Albert Einstein

Most books on health focus solely on diet and exercise. This book goes further, providing a compass that helps the reader connect to nature and use those energetic connections to navigate a path to a more vibrant and happier life. It offers simple practices the reader can develop into habits without any expensive supplements, gym memberships, or techno-gizmos. For most people, these simple practices will not even necessitate permission from a health care practitioner, as they pose no medical risk.

These practices also work to sustain us as a population and a species. Not only do they have the potential to heal us personally, but also following them works to mitigate, or even repair, the very human activities that threaten all contemporary life with ecological and political crisis.

I have spent four decades working as an occupational therapy clinician, treating people of all ages, from infants to centenarians. I have worked with people who suffered catastrophic accidents and devastating chronic disease. As occupational therapists we help people develop habits that transform their lives, habits so small they sometimes get overlooked by others. Occupational therapists define *occupation* more broadly than most people. We work on any and all activities, including the five occupations that form the framework of this book—playing, sleeping, eating, working, and loving (American Occupational Therapy Association, Inc., 2017).

Although I felt firmly grounded in conventional Western medicine, when some patients began telling me of their experiences with traditional folk heal-ers I saw similarities with occupational therapy. Not only did traditional healers focus on seemingly mundane details, like getting dressed or cooking a meal, but they used very sensory-dense treatments that sounded much like *sensory integration*, an innovative neurological approach focused on changing the entire nervous system through movement, touch, vision, hearing, smell, and taste. The sensory integration approach often produced amazing results with children who had learning disabilities, ADHD, and autism.

From my perspective it seemed as if traditional healers had been using neu-rosensory techniques for millennia, and I wanted to take a closer look. In those days before integrative, functional, or holistic medicine became popular, Harvard Divinity School provided me with an opportunity to explore these ideas.

In the decades following my graduation from Harvard, the study of physics, epigenetics, evolutionary biology, neurophysiology, and immunology has made quantum leaps, and these fields all support the traditional healer concept: the belief in our phenomenal ability to grow and recover from unimaginable trau-mas and dysfunction. It often seems to me that our science has finally caught up to truths traditional healers have known forever. Their low-tech approach to healing has always made it sustainable, relying more on energetic practices than complex technology-dependent evaluation tools, invasive operations, and expensive pharmaceuticals..

Beliefs create thoughts.
Thoughts create emotions.
Emotions create actions.
Actions create health.

If we *believe* that our body is like a machine with parts that break down we may *think* that nothing we do personally can cause any kind of lasting change. We *fear* aches and pains. We *worry* about getting old. We listen to advertise-ments that promise relief and eternal youth, even if those same advertisements warn us that these products could cause serious side effects.

If we *believe* our body speaks to us in signs and symptoms telling us what it needs, then we will take time to listen and *question* what we can do to get back into harmony. We feel *love* for how our bodies constantly heal and repair them-selves, and we do what we can to encourage and support our health.

If we hold the first set of beliefs, we may feel our only option puts us at the mercy of a system that entails costly technological interventions, ones that may produce near-miraculous results but stand wholly outside of our own ability to intervene on behalf of our own health.

Holding the second set of beliefs, we become the stewards of our own lives. The power of healing rests in our own hands. We may consult others whose knowledge is greater than our own, whether conventional medical practitioners or traditional healers. This second set of beliefs also provides us with many more low-cost or even free ways we can act to improve our own health.

The Healing Compass of Sustainable Health can serve as a guide to beginning a conversation with our bodies. In doing so, we need to hold awareness of our minds' role in these conversations. Our minds tell us stories. These stories pull together information from our beliefs and emotions, weaving explanations borne of both logic and intuition, though not necessarily truth. For truth we need a spiritual connection with the natural world and the chance to observe natural laws at work. For truth we need to listen to our body as it speaks to us in sensations and emotions.

When people speak of integrative or functional medicine, they often talk about body, mind, and spirit, but spirit can get lost as we focus on the physical reality of the body and the countless stories that come to us from science, literature, religious doctrine, and popular media. We can best hear the voice of spirit in nature and in the still moments we have when our consciousness connects with the consciousness of the universe through meditation or prayer. In that arena of infinite possibility, many kinds of healing can occur.

This book came out of a thought experiment, "How would my occupational therapy practice change if I followed traditional Chinese medicine (TCM) rather than a conventional Western medicine paradigm?"

Although most traditional healers pass their powerful wisdom from generation to generation orally through a few carefully selected students from within their own community, two traditions began writing their knowledge down about 2500 years ago. Most of us know yoga from the *Ayurveda* tradition of India and acupuncture from TCM. These two treatment techniques only represent a fraction of the traditions from whence they came. Nonetheless, they have both successfully made their way into conventional Western medicine. Many physicians, nurses, and other health professionals have incorporated yoga and acupuncture into their practices, even though these originated from spiritual and energy-based approaches. They use these techniques because they provide positive outcomes such as amelioration or even reversal of symptoms for their patients. Both yoga and acupuncture have become so accepted that many corporate wellness programs and even insurance companies reimburse for their use in treatment.

TCM approaches patients in a way that is very compatible with occupational therapy practice. Both kinds of practitioners focus on what people can do, as well as how they feel about the world around them, the people in their lives, and their dreams for a future. They listen to their patients' stories, observe how they move, and consider their reactions to all aspects of their environment. TCM understands the power of sensory processing and daily activities in healing in much the same way occupational therapists do.

Although occupational therapy recognizes the importance of spirituality, spirituality does not infuse our practice in the same way it does in TCM. This book will connect body, mind, and spirit through TCM's Five Element Theory, which focuses on natural laws that govern energetic interactions between the elements of Wood, Water, Earth, Metal, and Fire. The Healing Compass that forms the basis for Sustainable Health comes out of this tradition.

Some people reading this book may find any discussions of spirit or soul disconcerting. Others may find the book's spiritual grounding in evolution and cos-

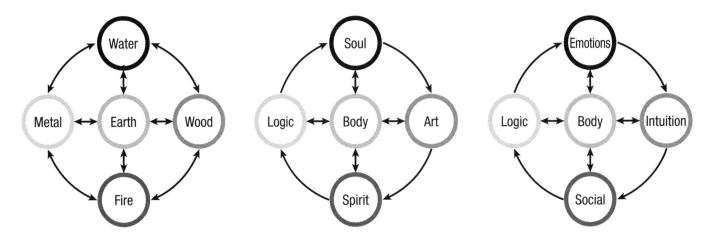

Figure 0.1   The Healing Compass takes elements from Traditional Chinese Medicine's Five Element Theory and relates these to Body, Mind, and Spirit approaches used by Holistic, Integrative, and Functional Medicine. The body's health depends on using the logical and artistic, intuitive mind as well as the social and emotional connections we make with others.

mology at variance with their own religious belief systems. I would hope that all readers, regardless of their orientation, take what helps their bodies, intrigues their minds, and connects them more closely to their own sense of spirit and soul so that they may benefit from the practices outlined in this book.

Ken Wilber, in his book, *The Marriage of Sense and Soul: Integrating Science and Religion*, makes a case for letting go of the stories that undergird all religions, in favor of examining the practices they espouse. He asks religious people to suspend belief for a time, for the simple reason that if *one* creation story becomes the *one* truth, then thousands of other stories become false. He asks scientists to participate in spiritual practices and hold them to the same standard of replicable results they would ask of other scientific observations. He asks us all to take a moment to look through Galileo's telescope before condemning his conclusion that we are not the center of the known universe. I feel we could all benefit from acknowledging such a change in perspective, for our own health as well as for that of the life forms that surround us.

At the time of my theological study in the early 1980s, integrative medicine had not entered the lexicon. Only people on the fringes of academia and medicine talked about body, mind, and spirit. The medical community held these practices in disregard, at best explaining positive outcomes as placebo effects. Over the following three decades, scientific discoveries and theories have explained many of these disregarded approaches.

Quantum physics and mechanics describe the interrelationship of energy and matter on the level of atoms and subatomic particles. At these levels matter behaves less and less like our world dominated by gravity, a world we have come to understand through Newton's laws. We all find a world where we can predict outcomes comforting. Beginning in the early 20th century, quantum physics and quantum mechanics radically disturbed our sense of predictable reality. When Einstein wrote the equation $E = mc^2$, he opened the door to a whole new understanding of matter and energy, one that depended on our point of observation in a continuum of space and time that we no longer visualized as linear. We came to understand that once particles connect they can still affect each other even at great distances. Niels Bohr, the Nobel Prize–winning physicist, put the Chinese symbol of yin and yang on his coat of arms because it represented his theory of complementarity. Indeed, physics began to sound more and more like spiritual teachings that connect everything in the universe.

Evolutionary biology has benefited greatly from discoveries from the field of epigenetics, which describes how our environment affects genetic expression and explains why the ways we play, sleep, eat, work, and love make us both unique and similar. The connections they have made between infinite arrays of species embody the interconnected complementarity described in physics.

In neuroscience, our understanding of neuroplasticity describes the myriad ways our brains and nervous systems find to reorganize and develop new connections and even new neurons. These understandings explain how people can recover from and compensate for serious injury, disease, and changes in our environment. Neuroscience has opened up whole new avenues of pharmacologic, surgical, and therapeutic realms of intervention in rehabilitation.

Immunology has introduced us to the ecosystems we carry within our bodies and how they help us stay healthy despite particular genetic markers. Immunology often explains how we can reverse what we once thought of as incurable diseases.

Even the placebo effect has been shown to have as much or more power than biomedical substrates used in pharmaceuticals (Rutherford, 2013). A growing number of physicians have made meditation practices central to their treatment of physical health problems (Brogan, 2016; Hyman, 2016; Siegel, 2016).

Our lives begin with our first inspiration and end with our last. Along the way we develop habits. Those habits change us in every imaginable way. As an occupational therapist, I know the power of changing one simple habit at a time. I know they accumulate and get stronger with practice. As a theologian and spiritual practitioner, I have had to learn patience. Miracles happen every day in occupational therapy. Many of them creep up slowly and catch us by surprise. The Healing Compass has helped me and my clients develop habits that set a course for health and happiness.

I believe that we have untapped power to heal ourselves. With this book I hope to share with readers a Healing Compass to help them take charge of their health and happiness, one habit, one day, one miracle at a time.

SUSTAINABLE HEALTH

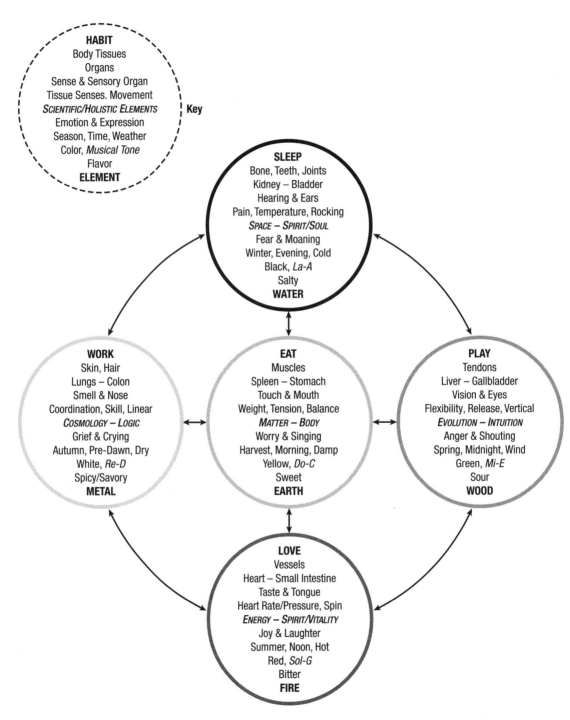

Figure 1.1 The Healing Compass and its Elemental associations. Each of the five elements has specific characteristics related to their elemental energy profile.

CHAPTER 1

Introduction to Sustainable Health

Using a Healing Compass

The body heals with play, the mind heals with laughter,
and the spirit heals with joy.

—PROVERB

SUSTAINABLE HEALTH MEANS taking charge of our own health. It also means feeling more at home in our own skin, loving our bodies, and loving this marvelous blue planet we call home.

It turns out that when we begin taking care of ourselves, we also take care of our immediate surroundings, as well as the places and people who matter in our lives. Our experience, intuition, and no shortage of scientific research tell us that the ever-growing soup of environmental toxins produced by our way of life has triggered an increase in chronic disease. Environmental toxins have been implicated in autism, Alzheimer's, cancer, depression, diabetes, heart disease, multiple sclerosis, obesity, and Parkinson's (Schauss, 2015).

We worry about our health, and we worry about how much it will cost us to stay healthy. According to a 2016 report from the Centers for Medicare and Medicaid Services, the United States spends almost 20% of its Gross Domestic Product on health care. In 2017 the National Center for Health Statistics reported that our yearly per person total health care expenditures have risen from $125 in 1960 to $8,468 in 2015. The Organisation for Economic Co-Operation and Development noted that the United States spends twice as much on health care as Canada, and U.S. citizens pay almost five times more than Canadian citizens do. U.S. citizens have good reason to worry about the costs of staying healthy.

We get plenty of advice about preventing disease through lifestyle choices:

Get exercise, sleep 8 hours a night, eat organic foods, and reduce stress. We know exercise is important, but gym memberships cost money and time. Supplements, such as vitamins, minerals, and all manner of health-touting food additives, protein shakes, and energy bars also cost plenty—and have very mixed results in clinical trials for their effectiveness, if they have had any verifiable testing at all. Organic produce and meats generally cost about three times more than conventional grocery store products.

We get bombarded by overwhelmingly bad news about a multitude of threats to our health, and we often feel powerless to do anything meaningful to change it. Stress mounts while sleep, work, and relationships suffer. Advertising often delivers the worst news. It used to be said that advertisers marketed everything to us through the enticement of sex. Maybe so in the past, but nowadays marketing seems to revolve around *fear.* So much advertising has fear at its core. Fear of not having enough money, charm, friends, or time. As a result, we invest in beauty enhancers, social media apps that connect us with other people, and labor-saving devices to give us more time.

The scariest advertising of all threatens us with illness. When we read the fine print or listen to the end of the commercial we learn that the pharmaceuticals promoted may kill us or make us sicker than the disease it says it cures.

Sometimes it seems as if we live our lives in a sea of fear that drains us of energy, ramps up our stress hormones, and sets off a host of inflammatory processes throughout our bodies. Scientists have determined that stress and inflammation can overwhelm our genetic resistance to fend off tissue damage or the current crop of seasonal pathogens (McEwen, 2008, 2012).

We used to think we couldn't do anything about genetics, but once scientists mapped out the human genome they found that we had more diseases than genes to cause them. Then researchers took a closer look and discovered our genes spark on and off like lightning bugs on a summer night. We would need a whole lot of them to stay on, all at the same time, to read a book. Now scientists want to know what processes trigger those flashes, what causes them to stay lit, what quiets them down, and how we pass those genes on to our offspring, either lit up or dormant. We call this field of science the study of *epigenetics.*

Like seeds in the ground, genes need just the right combinations of environmental factors to flourish. Although plenty of research money pours into epigenetics research, we already know a couple of simple things that cause genes to express themselves. We don't have to wait for undiscovered drugs or fancy technology to activate our genes, because we have evidence that food and relief from stress will do the job.

We have at our disposal these two very important genetic change agents. If we feed our body what it needs to stay healthy and change our habits to reduce our stress levels, we can stay healthy and happier longer. Our personal application of epigenetics affects emotions and mood as well as bodily processes.

When we reduce stress, we reduce inflammation. When we reduce inflammation, our bodies heal. Do we worry that scratch we got shaving won't heal? No. Unless we have some very dangerous medical condition, we know our cells will rapidly mobilize, and in minutes blood will stop oozing. In an hour we will have a protective scab and in a few days that scab will drop off and reveal brand new skin. Although we can't see them, the same processes work inside our bodies. We need to learn how to trust those processes again.

Beliefs create thoughts.
Thoughts create emotions.
Emotions create actions.
Actions create health.

If we *believe* that everything that can help us stay healthy depends on cutting-edge technology and pharmaceuticals, we *think* that we will need lots of money to stay well. We will *worry* about insurance premiums, co-pays, and the choices politicians or insurance executives make behind closed doors. We may feel at turns both *angry* and *helpless*. No wonder some of us seek temporary relief in a box of doughnuts, a bottle of pills, shopping malls, casinos, or simply a margarita or three.

If we *believe* our body has innate powers of adaptation, self-regulation, and the ability to create new cells to replace the damaged ones, we *realize* it does this every second of every day we breathe. Worry diminishes as fear and anger dissipate. We feel *empowered* to support those processes.

The Healing Compass that forms the core of Sustainable Health can provide us with a tool to lead us away from overwhelming feelings of helplessness, back to a sense of feeling in control again. It puts our health back into our own hands.

Our journey to Sustainable Health—that is, feeling good and staying well without all sorts of supplements, techno-gizmos, and expensive treatments—relies on knowing which direction to take. Just as we would use a navigational compass to find our way on a journey, Sustainable Health uses a Healing Compass that orients us to our own needs and points us in directions we can follow. Our actions either lead us to improved health and well-being, or not.

Sustainable Health provides a road map of proven habits we can develop to bring us to healthier and happier lives. For many of us, health equates with weight loss. Indeed, obesity is epidemic around the world, and weight loss unquestionably produces improved health outcomes for most people, but for several reasons this book describes a journey to health and happiness, not weight loss.

It's not just about the weight. About 30% of obese people have perfectly good health in spite of their weight. They have normal cholesterol, blood sugar, and other metabolic parameters. Plenty of skinny people have metabolic problems like diabetes, cardiovascular disease, and cancer. Indeed, people with metabolic healthy obesity (MHO) seem to have mortality rates similar to those who have normal body weights and body mass index (BMI) (Satter, 2017).

Weight loss is a complex, multidimensional issue. As any of us who have ever attempted weight loss can say, for most of us it results in short-term losses and long-term gains (in pounds). We are born with a finite number of fat cells, depending on our genetics as well as our mother's lifestyle during her pregnancy. We can fill or not fill those cells, but we can't get rid of fat cells with anything short of surgery or other destructive medical procedures.

Our bodies will do everything they can to maintain weight and nurture fat cells. For most of our three million or so years as a species, we have had to cope with famine far more often than with the daily feast of meals and snacks we enjoy today. Chapter 4: Earth Energies, will cover eating and weight in more depth, because scientists have begun to regard fat as an organ that plays a major role in our hormone levels as well as our immune responses (Tara, 2017).

Despite this caveat about weight loss, every one of the habits on our journey to Sustainable Health has a proven track record with weight loss and many other health parameters. Sustainable Health means befriending our bodies, minds, and spirits. It means surrendering to the wisdom of Mother Nature and enjoying the scenery as we travel along this journey called life. We are not machines made up of parts. We more closely resemble a universe made up of vast numbers of species and environments. We appear to carry more DNA for the microorganisms that inhabit us than we do for our own cells. Most of our cells, as well as the species who call us home, have our best interests at heart. They usually work for us, not against us. Our spiritual connections, our beliefs, and our physiology have no real demarcations other than those we have constructed with our thoughts and feelings.

Healing versus Curing with Meditation and Other Alternative Practices

Many people begin a meditation or other alternative health practice because they hope to reverse the symptoms of disease. Indeed, research has shown a surprisingly reliable reduction of symptoms for a great many people with a variety of practices, from meditation to supplements. We may say that these people have been "cured," however most alternative health practitioners prefer the term "healing." Healing lets go of our attachment to the outcome. It keeps us focused on the present moment. Awareness, breathing, observation, movement, eating, and gratitude practices allow us to transcend outcome and realize the preciousness of what we experience day to day. By accepting our present circumstances and trusting our body's innate wisdom, all experiences—pain, joy, sadness, anger, fear, anxiety—come and go. We no longer feel trapped and can accept our situation with grace and dignity.

Have Faith

When I give seminars on healing I often hand each participant a tiny mustard seed to illustrate faith's role in our natural ability to heal, whether from a small cut or a serious diagnosis. If you take that tiny seed and put it on a bit of dirt in a warm sunny spot, and give it regular rations of water, it will grow into a large weedy plant full of nutrients. If you let that plant flower, it will provide enough seeds to plant a whole field of greens. Plant those seeds at midsummer, and within a month, from that single seed, you can provide enough greens for a whole family.

Many participants lose their tiny seed before we even finish the seminar. Like tiny seeds, faith gets easily lost. Like tiny seeds, faith occurs in abundance, and you can find plenty more. Provide a seed with dirt, sun, and water to transform energy into nourishment.

Think of this journey as a seed. It grows when you provide it time and space. Without these basic requirements it withers. Don't hold on to regrets. Let them go. Find another seed. Start again another day. Health, happiness, and seeds all grow in abundance.

Approach this journey as a scientist studying your own body, mind, and spirit. N = 1 is scientific jargon for a study of one person or subject. Try each habit described in this book, and watch what happens in your own life. Perhaps you will achieve a weight you only dreamed possible. Maybe you will wake up without the allergies that have plagued you since childhood or realize a painful joint no longer bothers you. Healing is in your hands, and possibilities abound!

Science and Spirit: Beliefs Behind the Healing Compass of Sustainable Health

Our journey starts by examining what we believe about our own ability to heal based on myths and science. We often interpret the stories ancient and indigenous people tell to explain the natural world as myths. These stories imbue natural phenomena with personalities and characteristics that explain their behavior. For instance, *Oya*, the Yoruba goddess of winds, lightning, and violent storms, swirls into life through tornadoes and hurricanes. As an unstoppable warrior, she governs change, the marketplace, life, and death (Gleason, 1992). Each detail of her many stories has some bit of wisdom that helps those who are caught up in stormy weather, or stormy relationships, understand their experience.

Science tells stories about our natural world with the details spelled out through mathematic equations and theories, devoid of emotional drama. Science can further our understanding of storms and other natural phenomena without ever contradicting the poetry and symbolism of myth. Both forms make up useful human belief systems.

To begin our healing journey, we must let go of a powerful story that shapes our everyday life. Most of us believe that our society and culture has reached the pinnacle of human development. Archaeology and anthropology do not bear this out. We have patchy information about how ancient civilizations constructed the pyramids, Machu Picchu, Stonehenge, or the Easter Island monoliths. Many forgotten civilizations had writing and all manner of technologies we have lost and cannot replicate. They did this without the immense amounts of energy provided by fossil fuels or nuclear fission, through their ingenuity, labor, and animal assistance. I will always remember Neil Armstrong's first step on the moon, and I can appreciate the value of vaccines, since I have met and treated people forever damaged by polio and rubella. Unfortunately, our use of fossil fuel-based technologies has unquestionably contributed to vast destruction of our planet's diverse ecosystems and threatens human health, as well.

Ancient healers understood the universe as interconnected, conscious relationships between natural elements. Healers developed intuitive practices based on these relationships and used them to move energy and transform matter. Most traditions organize these observations into four or more elements placed around geomagnetic directional points on a compass. Each tradition develops stories which represent these elements through a variety of mythic characters. Stories explain the relationships between these characters, enabling people to predict how the elements will behave under different conditions.

People often represent these associations with a cross enclosed in a circle. This symbol crops up around the globe in various media, such as pictographs carved in stone, designs in jewelry, paintings, and other objects in daily use.

The earliest compasses found in Chinese and Mesoamerican archaeological sites date back two to three thousand years. They appear to have been used by orienting to the magnetic poles for healing or *feng shui* types of activities (Carlson, 1975; Guimarães, 2004). The use of a compass as a navigational

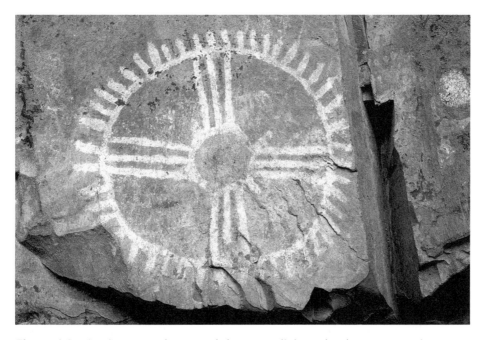

Figure 1.2 Ancient people carved these medicine wheel compasses into rocks all over the North American Southwest, like this Palatki Sun Shield from Sedona, Arizona.

tool came later, dating back only a thousand years. Becoming mindful of these ancient implements for organizing the natural world through complementary spiritual and material concepts allows us to explore a unique path to healing.

For most of the past three million years of human existence on this planet, everyone from toddler to elder has known the basic navigation of sunrise (East) and sunset (West) as a means for finding one's way home. In the past century of indoor living and 24-hour work schedules, we have lost our orientation to the natural world. Many of us can no longer identify the cardinal points of North, South, East, and West without a directional finder. We can fly around the planet in a matter of days. We know that humans have traveled to the moon and back. Could we find our way home from an unfamiliar place without our trusty satellite navigation applications? The Healing Compass serves as a physical and spiritual road map, a guide to our place on this beautiful planet.

My studies of healing traditions at Harvard led me to many different versions of the Healing Compass. Each one organized information around the directional points in slightly different variations passed on orally from generation to generation. The placement of the elements around a circle relied on geographic and cultural understandings unique to each tradition. Over the years I have con-

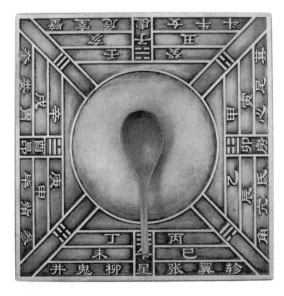

Figure 1.3 This early Chinese compass used a spoon made of magnetic lodestone placed on a board that showed the geomagnetic directions and their associations. It was used for healing and *feng shui* types of activities during the 2nd through 4th centuries BCE, and did not find its way into navigation until many centuries later.

structed my own Healing Compasses according to several different traditions. Natural elements move around the cardinal points and get associated with different properties, while still retaining a fundamental method of organizing complex elements into a simple paradigm for healing.

For several reasons, in Sustainable Health we will use a configuration based on Five Element Theory from TCM. It comes to us from an unbroken lineage that goes back for many thousands of years, including more than two thousand years of written documentation. The five elements and their compass points originated with Taoist principles regarding natural phenomena (Lu & Schaplowsky, 2015). These feel more compatible with modern science than those compasses derived from the interaction of gods, goddesses, and spirits.

The Healing Compass of Sustainable Health uses five basic elements: Earth, Wood, Metal, Water, and Fire. Our Healing Compass employs this configuration based on thousands of years of observation. When capitalized, these words indicate the properties associated with these elements from TCM's Five Element Theory, rather than their everyday use in language.

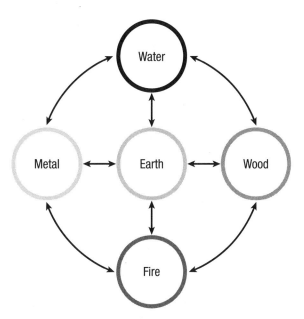

Figure 1.4   The Five Elements of Traditional Chinese Medicine placed in their position on a magnetic compass with North at the top. These designations come from traditional correspondences.

Five Element Theory organizes these elements according to the cardinal (geomagnetic) points of a compass in the following arrangement:

- Earth in the center
- Wood to the East
- Metal to the West
- Water to the North
- Fire to the South.

We can also view the Healing Compass from the belief system of contemporary science, and the four elements of Energy, Matter, Time, and Space. Physics, chemistry, and biology have much to offer for understanding these natural elements. Scientific study has taken great steps forward since the beginning of the 20th century. Prior to the last century, science measured only what could be discerned through our five discriminative senses, using increasingly complex machines such as microscopes and telescopes. As Einstein and others ushered in a new era of subatomic exploration, the technology got more complex and the observations got weirder, sounding more and more fantastic, and more similar to descriptions from traditional healers. Both scientists and traditional healers understand the universe through observation and replicable results to back up new theories and perspectives. When capitalized, the terms Energy, Matter, Space, and Time indicate our scientific understanding rather than colloquial definitions.

- Matter in the center
- Biological Time or Evolution to the East
- Cosmological Time or Big Bang theory to the West
- Space to the North
- Energy to the South.

In our Healing Compass, Energy, the ability to do work, resonates with Fire. Although we think of fire as thermal energy, in the context of our Healing Compass it will include all forms of energy, including both kinetic (movement) and potential (stored). Some of these forms of Energy resonate strongly with other elements in the compass. For instance, sound, a form of mechanical energy, and color, from the visible spectrum of electromagnetic radiation, have expression in all of the elements.

Matter corresponds with Earth. It takes up space and responds to forces of gravity that we can measure quite accurately thanks to Sir Isaac Newton's observations more than three centuries ago. Newton's laws laid the groundwork of physics for almost 250 years prior to the new understandings that emerged from Einstein's general theory of relativity. In the Healing Compass, Earth also includes all things of this planet, including us and the soil, where life took root after emerging from the sea. Earth also corresponds to elements of Matter, like organs and tissues, found in each element of the Healing Compass.

Time, as Einstein elegantly pointed out, is relative. Physicists tell many varied and complex mathematic stories about time. In the Healing Compass we have two stories about Time. As Metal we refer to cosmological time, the Big Bang, and the spread of "stardust" throughout the known universe. We think in terms of sky, stars, and planets, including the chemical elements from the periodic table that formed our planet. As Wood we tell a story of evolution, the amazing diversity of life both seen and unseen. Both evolution and cosmologic time unfold over extremely long periods. We also have a more personal way to view time, measured by seasons and hours of the day and night. These shorter time periods correspond with each element of the Healing Compass.

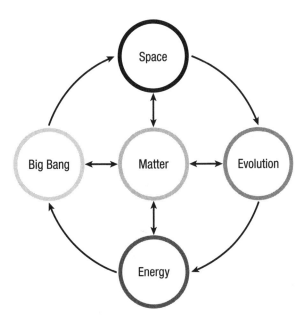

Figure 1.5 Five Elements from Science – Energy, Matter, Space and Time. Time depends on the perspective of the observer. Physicists tell us about the Big Bang Theory while biologists tell us about evolution.

Space connects us to the farthest reaches of the universe. Space, like Water, remains a largely unexplored mystery. Physicists have spent a lot of effort trying to figure out the composition of the universe. Some, like Peter Russell, author of *From Science to God: A Physicist's Journey into the Mystery of Consciousness,* have begun to speak about a universe composed of consciousness. This explanation comes closer to the notions of theologians and indigenous healers.

Physicists tell us that Time and Space cannot be separated, and as soon as we examine Matter from the viewpoint of science, we see that it also contains more Space than actual stuff. Indeed, science tells us that the three familiar forms of Matter (that is, gases, liquids, and solids) differ in the strength of their energetic bonds and the space between molecules. As physicists drill down deeper and deeper, molecules become atoms, atoms become particles, and eventually even those particles disappear and it's all energetic waves.

A scientific poet might describe us as collections of stardust solidified by myriads of energetic bonds, held to the earth through the invisible power of gravity, which dances in concert with the sun and moon, ever growing and diversifying, in infinite cycles of life, death, life . . .

Einstein put it like this: $E = mc^2$. Energy and Matter become the same thing in nature, which holds speed (space divided by time) constant at the speed of light squared. Fluidity between Energy and Matter and the inseparability of Time and Space opened up whole new worlds for scientists.

Sensations, Thoughts, and Emotions: The Mind's Confusing Twists and Turns

We like to make sense of our world, so we make up stories about all the information that comes to us from our senses. Throughout our lives, we build up memories about what we have seen, heard, touched, smelled, and tasted— what happened that we associate with those sensations, and the emotions that accompanied them. We interpret thoughts through our beliefs and act on the stories we make up to explain these combinations of beliefs, thoughts, and emotions. Sometimes we get it quite accurately, and sometimes we don't. As we obtain new information, we can change our thoughts to accommodate

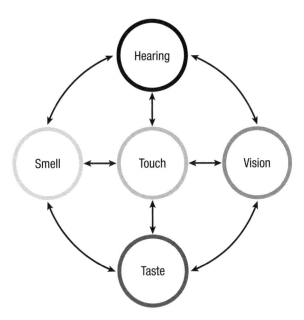

Figure 1.6 Five Element Compass for Our Discriminative Senses. Each sense has a traditional correspondence with an element and occurs on the compass in the position of that element.

that information or disregard it when it challenges a long-held and cherished belief system.

Our senses deliver information for us to remember and interpret. Each element of the Healing Compass resonates with a specialized sensory organ. These take in various kinds of energetic information.

Light: Electromagnetic Radiation

Our eyes sense light intensity and color. Light travels rapidly through Space And Time and comes to us in waves of electromagnetic radiation, measured by Space, nanometers (nm), and Time, Terahertz (THz) a description of frequency. Objects that absorb or reflect these waves appear to us as colors. Some of those waves register as colors we can "see" only through technology, such as infrared and ultraviolet light. Colors associated with various elements appear on the Healing Compass. Think about your favorite colors, the clothes you wear, the paint on the walls, and the colors you see in nature. Find them on the Healing Compass. We often choose colors to support our health and our feelings about ourselves and the world around us. Here they are from longest to shortest wavelength.

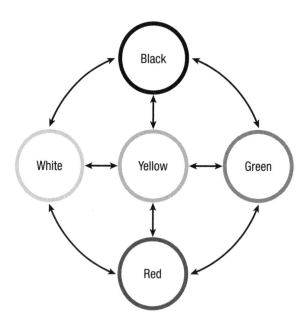

Figure 1.7 Five Element Color Compass – Light Energy. Each color has a traditional correspondence with an element and occurs on the compass in the position of that element.

- Yellow (590–560 nm/510–540 THz) in the center
- Green (560–520 nm/540–580 THz) to the East
- Red (700–635 nm/430–480 THz) to the South
- White (scatters all wavelengths) to the West
- Black (absorbs all wavelengths) to the North.

Wood resonates with the eyes and vision. Plants absorb all light wavelengths but green. Some people also associate Wood with the color blue (490–450 nm/610–670 THz). Plants grow on Earth (yellow) which mixes with blue to make green. Red has the longest wavelength we can see. Longer wavelengths generate more heat than shorter wavelengths and we associate the color red with Fire.

White light contains all the colors of the visible spectrum or reflects them back to us in the objects we see as white. We see the moon, stars, and planets as white because of the way our eyes work, but sensitive equipment can pick up smaller variations than we can see. Many animals can see wavelengths we can't.

Black absorbs all the wavelengths of visible light, just as deep water and black jeans do. You can feel the heat of that absorbed light through your clothes. Black holes in space absorb all light, and the blackness we see between stars covers the light of stars whose light has not yet traveled to us.

Sound: Mechanical Energy

Sound comes to us through mechanical waves that move our tympanic membranes, also known as eardrums. Our ears have bones which help to conduct these sound waves. Each element in the Healing Compass has a specific tone (wavelength) from the pentatonic scale associated with it.

Studies have shown that our brain waves will synchronize to sound waves (Doelling & Poeppel, 2015). Many different cultures base music on a five-note (pentatonic) scale where all the tones harmonize. A pentatonic scale lacks discordant notes, so it soothes and calms us.

If you have ever watched the movie or musical, *The Sound of Music*, you have some passing familiarity with the *do, re, mi (solfège)* terms of music education. The frequency intervals of *solfège* mean you can move these notes into any key and still maintain the mathematic or frequency ratio, which shortens as the notes go higher and lengthens as the notes go lower. The Healing Compass shows solfège intervals using notes from the C major scale.

- *Do* in the center, associated with Earth and middle C on a piano keyboard
- *Re* to the West, associated with Metal and D on the piano

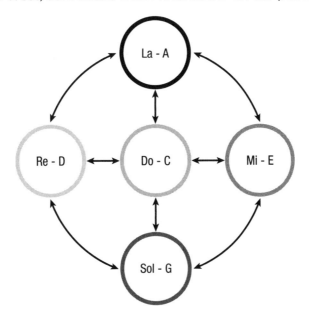

Figure 1.8 Five Element Sound Compass – Mechanical Energy. Each note has a traditional correspondence with an element and occurs on the compass in the position of that element.

- *Mi* to the East, associated with Wood and E on the piano
- *Sol* to the South, associated with Fire and G on the piano
- *La* to the North, associated with Water and A on the piano.

Each note in music resonates with mechanical energy, and since most music uses a wide range of notes we can see how it can play a powerful a role in healing. Many indigenous healers sing or chant over their patients. Contemporary sound healers from industrialized societies use both musical instruments and technology to produce these waves.

Touch and Movement: Mechanical, Gravitational, and Kinetic Energies
We explore our world through our senses of touch and movement. Our skin is full of all sorts of specialized nerve endings that can sense pain, temperature, and various kinds of pressure. The lips, tongue, thumb, fingers, toes, and feet have the densest concentrations of these receptors. We also have sensory receptors in muscles, tendons, joints, and blood vessels. Because we constantly move in relationship to the earth's gravity, we have a very important organ called the vestibular apparatus deep inside our inner ear that tells us exactly how we move in relation to the earth's gravitational forces. Our vestibular system has multiple

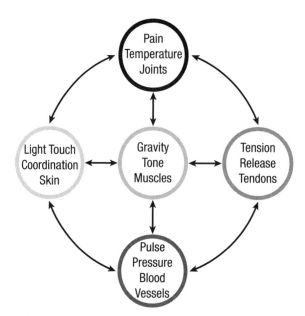

Figure 1.9 Five Element Body Tissue Sensations – Kinesthesia and Proprioception. Each body tissue provides sensory information. The tissues correspond with the elements and occur on the compass in the position of that element.

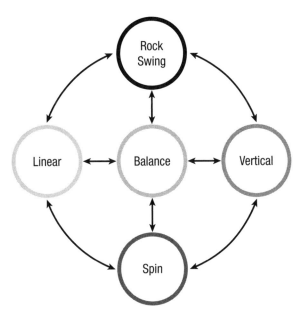

Figure 1.10   Five Element Movement Sensations – Vestibular System. Each direction of movement corresponds to ways we discern movement. I have taken the liberty of associating these movements with how each of the Five Elements behaves in nature, and linking them to that element's traditional position on the compass.

connections to other parts of our brain. It regulates our balance and all sorts of movements and even emotions. These receptors for touch and movement work in synchrony and guide us in multiple, complex ways. We will cover these in more detail throughout this book.

Taste and Smell: Chemical Energy

Our noses have elaborate receptors that allow us to make almost immediate chemical analysis of scents. Our noses once directed us to find food and water, though now we usually use our eyes and ears to respond to advertising and health claims. Our sense of smell can warn us of danger or attract us to a mate. Our sense of taste also makes chemical analyses, aided to a great degree by our sense of smell. Each point on the Healing Compass has a specific flavor associated with it.

- Earth, in the center, resonates with the sweet flavors of fruits
- Wood, to the East, resonates with the sour flavors of plants
- Metal, in the West, resonates with spicy or savory flavors
- Water, in the North, resonates with the salty flavor of oceans
- Fire, in the South, resonates with bitter flavors, like charred food.

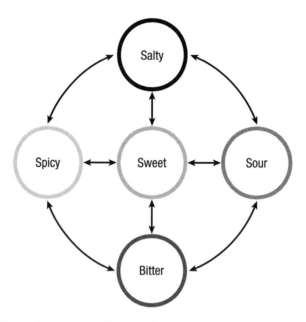

Figure 1.11 The Flavor Compass – Chemical Energy. Each flavor has a correspondence with an element and occurs on the compass in the position of that element.

Emotions

Our mind takes sensations and coordinates them with emotions. Memory helps us remember which events and sensations led to stressful, dangerous emotions and which events and sensations led to pleasurable and happy emotions. Five emotions have a place in the Healing Compass. Each of these emotions has a function, and they need to work in harmony. When we suppress one, it finds other avenues of expression, often in physical symptoms.

- Worry, in the center, resonates with Earth and our mind's all too frequent tendency to overthink, ruminate, and obsess about things that interest us
- Anger, in the East, resonates with Wood and the relentless drive to grow and thrive
- Grief, in the West, resonates with Metal and our sadness over inevitable losses we can't control
- Fear, in the North, resonates with Water and the depths of what we don't yet know
- Joy, in the South, resonates with Fire that lights up our nights and warms our hearts.

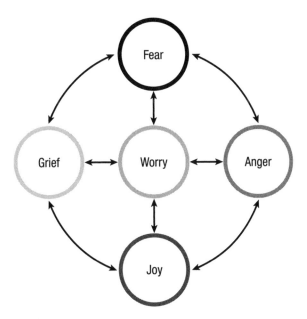

Figure 1.12 Five Element Emotions Compass. Each emotion has a correspondence with an element and occurs on the compass in the position of that element.

Our thoughts and emotions can guide us, but our bodies always tell the truth about suppressed emotions (Miller, 2005). The Healing Compass can help guide our actions.

The Body Never Lies: Actions Create Health

The Healing Compass relies on our physical world to orient our minds. We may tell ourselves all kinds of stories, but what we feel in our bodies forms our deepest and most reliable guide.

- Wood, to the East, resonates with tendons and our ability to be flexible when stressed. Our livers and gallbladders play a part in detoxifying all kinds of stressors, both physical and mental. Our eyes depend on flexibility for focus and clarity. Play relieves stress; Chapter 2's focus on Play will introduce a practice that relieves stress by using our eyes to enjoy and appreciate the ever-changing life around us.
- Water, to the North, resonates with bones, teeth, and joints that connect us to protective, if unpleasant, experiences of pain when we go against

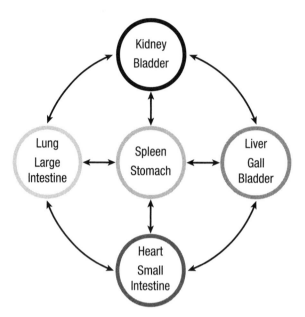

Figure 1.13 Five Element Organs Compass. Each pair of organs has a correspondence with an element and occurs on the compass in the position of that element.

the flow of what our bodies need to stay healthy. Our kidneys and bladder help us manage water content in our bodies. We may use heat or cold to manage painful body parts or soothe ourselves by listening to music and rocking. Sleep heals us on deep levels within our brains and bodies. Chapter 3's focus on Sleep introduces a practice that confronts fear and promotes restful, healing sleep.

- Earth, in the center, resonates with muscles and our use of force to overcome the effects of gravity. Our stomach and spleen help us digest the food we eat, just as our minds work overtime to maintain mental and spiritual balance as we digest an overwhelming amount of information, coming to us from all kinds of media and our natural environment. We can try to regain our composure through food, but our sweet tooth often betrays us. Chapter 4's focus on Eating provides us with a new way of looking at food, concentrating on pleasure and debunking several long-held myths of dieting.

- Metal, to the West, resonates with skin and hair, often the harbingers of chemical toxicity or imbalance. Our lungs and colon help us release these toxins. We develop coordination by organizing the sensations of our skin moving over joints through repetition and practice (Greene & Roberts,

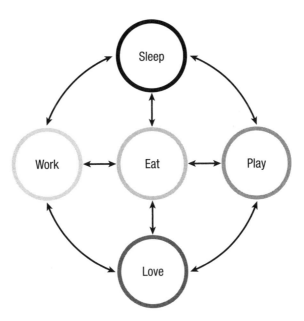

Figure 1.14   Five Element Occupations and Habits Compass. I have taken the liberty of associating these occupations with how each of the Five Elements behaves in nature, and linking them to that element's traditional position on the compass. Each chapter links these occupations to a specific practice that, with repetition, can become a habit that has a known potential to affect our health and happiness for the better.

2017). Chapter 5's focus on Work looks at a simple practice to detoxify our homes and ultimately the larger environment where we live and breathe.

- Fire, in the South, resonates with our heart and blood vessels, registering excitement and pressure. Our small intestine plays a part in heart health, and we all know there is no joy to be found when the gut is not happy! Laughter and enjoying the company of friends and family keeps our hearts healthy on both physical and spiritual planes. Chapter 6's focus on Love provides us with a practice to keep our lives joyful.

How to Use This Book

This journey to health and happiness offers a different path than most of us are familiar with using. While Sustainable Health considers the body, food, sleep, work, and many tangible acts and experiences of living, the power for producing results comes from energy, our own, and our ability to tap into the conscious energy of the world around us by connecting with nature. Each chapter asks us to examine our beliefs, thoughts, and emotions as we act to improve our health.

Take some time to look at the Healing Compass. Each chapter will cover the details associated with its element and provide a corresponding habit to bring our body, mind, and spirit back into harmony. To begin, think of the Healing Compass as a set of clues. Make note of aspects that affect your life right now. Do you have health problems with particular body tissues, organs, or senses? Do you find yourself troubled by certain emotions? Perhaps you don't recognize the emotion, but find yourself expressing it often with shouting, moaning, singing, crying, or laughing. Our contemporary society considers these symptoms things we need to correct. Sustainable Health turns that concept on its head. Our body communicates with the universe, even if we seem to have shut ourselves off from the natural world. These symptoms are clues to open up a dialogue. Rather than think of them as negatives to banish or correct, consider them as starting points in a conversation with your body and the natural world.

Our bodies constantly take care of us. They house our memories, experiences, and desires. Some might say they house our spirit and soul. Honor the amazing job that our bodies do digesting food, breathing, keeping blood flowing, and protecting us from dangers both seen and unseen.

Exercise 1.1: Get a Baseline Assessment of Health

Use the Sustainable Health Checklist to identify your health strengths and areas that could improve. The Sustainable Health Checklist focuses on health from a more conventional Western medicine perspective. Each section is arranged in five subsections to match the following five chapters, with those symptoms most likely to signal an issue arranged in Wood, Water, Earth, Metal, or Fire sequences. Scores of 4 or 5 in any area indicate health strengths, those aspects of health that support us. Scores of 3 signal a need to get into a serious conversation with our bodies about that area. Scores of 1 or 2 in any area mean that we might want to consider expanding that conversation to include a health care practitioner.

Worksheet 1.1: Sustainable Health Checklist

DAILY HABITS

SCORE	5	4	3	2	1
Outdoor Movement	Daily – sitting, bending, crawling, walking, running, jumping, climbing.		Daily – sitting, walking, bending, reaching.		Rarely if ever outdoors – due to pain, allergies, weakness, or fatigue.
Sleep	Average 7–9 hours/night – uninterrupted sleep – nap easily if tired.		Less than 8 hours/night – fitful nights – difficulty napping.		Inability to sleep more than a few hours at a time.
Mealtimes	Enjoy eating. Eat a variety of foods. Comfortable with food choices & availability.		Occasionally enjoy eating. Difficulties with food choices &/or availability.		Erratic eating. Strict food choices. Limited food choices &/or availability.
Work	Paid &/or unpaid work meaningful to you &/or others. Enjoy work life.		Paid &/or unpaid work essential to others. Work sometimes difficult or tedious.		No paid or unpaid work available. Self-care difficult to perform.
Social Interactions	Daily physical and face-to-face contact with people you love & enjoy.		Regular face-to-face contact with people you love & enjoy.		Rare or no face-to-face contact with people.

HABITS OF BELIEF

SCORE	5	4	3	2	1
Flexibility	I don't let things bother me. I go with the flow.		I follow the rules even if others don't.		I can't accept my own and/or others mistakes
Faith	I know everything always works for the best.		What goes around comes around.		I'm on my own in this world. No help expected.
Simplicity	Living is simple. I enjoy one day at a time.		I'd like to enjoy my days more but I'm too busy.		I'm usually overwhelmed just keeping up.
Gratitude	I wake up happy & thankful to be alive.		I work hard for what I have & I'm thankful.		It seems like other people have more than I do.
Love	I often say to myself, "what a wonderful life."		I find joy in my life with people I love.		I do what I can to get by.
Page Score:					

Worksheet 1.1: Sustainable Health Checklist *(continued)*

BODILY PROCESSES

SCORE	5	4	3	2	1
Detoxification **Skin**	Skin intact & supple.		Frequent skin eruptions-rashes, hives, pimples.		Chronic skin conditions require treatment.
Hair	Strong & shiny.		Dull, lifeless, brittle.		Unusual hair loss.
Nails	Smooth, hard, clear, good half-moons		Ridged, thin, brittle, spots, missing half-moons		Thick, broken, opaque.
Elimination **Bowel movements**	Brown, soft to firm consistency, 1-2 times/day.		Frequent hard stools, straining or loose stool, 1-2 times/week.		Infrequent, painful stools &/ or frequent diarrhea. Black or foul-smelling stools.
Urine	Usually clear or light yellow.		Frequently dark yellow.		Dark brown, red, orange, foul smell.
Sweat	Clear, salty, after active movement or getting hot		Rarely sweat even when warm or after exercise		Frequently sweat even when not active or in cool temperatures. Foul smell.
Digestion	Able to digest all foods without difficulty.		Cautious about food choices – allergies & sensitivities.		Chronic digestive disorders – IBS, Crohns, Celiac, or other GI issues.
Breathing	Breathe easily & deeply.		Congestion, difficulty breathing.		Cough, wheezing, asthma, lung disorders.
Cardiovascular	Enjoy an active lifestyle.		Difficulty breathing-discomfort when moving.		Chest pain. Getting treatment for heart disease.

MOVEMENT

SCORE	5	4	3	2	1
Flexibility	Able to reach overhead and to floor without difficulty.		Able to reach all parts of body for washing up and hygiene.		Need assistance to reach objects & body parts for washing up and hygiene.
Pain	Rarely troubled by pain.		Pain limits activities.		Pain limits movement.
Strength	Able to lift heavy objects. Regularly climb steps and/or ladders.		Need help for many tasks that involve lifting and climbing.		Never do any lifting or climbing.
Coordination	Learn skilled movements easily.		Need lots of practice to learn any new movement.		Clumsy, avoid most movement.
Stamina	Plenty of energy to get through the day.		Take frequent rest breaks.		More time spent resting than doing anything.
Page Score:					

SENSORY PROCESSING

SCORE	5	4	3	2	1
Vision	Eyes bright, shiny- normal vision.		Dark circles under eyes. Frequent tearing. Puffy, itchy eyes.		Blindness. Eye disorders and/ or diseases.
Hearing	Able to hear conversations in noisy environments		Tinnitus. Hearing loss. Occasional ear infections		Acute hearing loss. Frequent ear infections.
Touch	Enjoy touching, exploring textures, and being touched		Avoid certain textures and/or physical contact with others.		Avoid touching or being touched.
Smell	Aware of smells. Enjoy exploring smells.		Congestion, sneezing, and / or runny nose affect smell.		Unable to smell.
Taste	Enjoy exploring a variety of flavors.		Swelling of lips, tongue, mouth, & throat impairs ability to taste.		Unable to taste
Balance	Enjoy activities that challenge balance.		Occasional trips and falls.		Movement limited by dizziness and/or lack of balance.

MENTAL PROCESSES

SCORE	5	4	3	2	1
Mood	Generally alert, curious – go with the flow		Troubled by crises or events but recover in time		Daily upset with events, objects, people
Imagination/ Creativity	Make art, music, dance, food, crafts, or other creative activities daily.		Make art, music, dance, food, crafts, or other creative activities weekly.		Never make art, music, dance, food, crafts or other creative activities.
Self- Regulation	Generally comfortable in body and varied environments.		Frequent outbursts or withdrawal from activities.		Need medication to maintain emotional and/or physical status quo
Learning/ Problem Solving	Enjoy tackling new projects or problems.		Willing to try new things with support from others.		Avoid unfamiliar places, people or activities.
Empathy/ Compassion	Recognize other's emotions. Share and/or help others when possible.		Confused about other's emotions and/or how to help them.		Disinterested in other's emotions and/or how to help them.

Worksheet 1.1: Sustainable Health Checklist *(continued)*

EMOTIONS

SCORE	5	4	3	2	1
Anger	Generally, get mad and get over it quickly.		Frequently hold a grudge.		Often mad at the world.
Fear	Trust our own intuition to stay safe.		Frequently troubled by fearful news and advertising.		Avoid risks to the point of inaction
Anxiety	Interested in observing the world around us.		Frequently troubled by problems we want to fix.		Obsessed with problems that need fixing
Grief/ Depression	Able to cry when sad.		Unable to cry even when sad things happen.		Feel sad all the time.
Joy	Always wake up excited to start a new day.		Frequently laugh, smile, feel happy to be alive.		Use drugs, sex, & excitement to stay happy.
Page Score:					

Exercise 1.2: Assessing Elemental Health

The Healing Compass Clues Checklist takes a perspective more in line with a TCM approach. The Healing Compass Clues Checklist collects information related more specifically to the five elements. Finding lots of clues in one direction of the Healing Compass might point us toward focusing on the habit from that chapter as a starting point. When clues appear in most, or even all, directions of the Healing Compass, we might start at the beginning, read through each chapter, and try out that chapter's practice for a few days. We must commit to doing a practice for a month to get the full benefit of developing a habit. Start with the practice that feels right to you and your body.

Worksheet 1.2: Healing Compass Clues Checklist

Read through the table and circle or highlight behaviors you recognize in yourself. What areas seem to be in balance? What areas need attention? Celebrate your harmonies and understand they will always shift and change in a variety of ways. Try the Practices for those elements that seem to need more attention.

Behaviors *Healing Approach*	Deficient / Erratic *Nurture / Soothe*	What We Want to See *Harmony & Balance*	Excess / Stuck *Channel / Motivate*
WOOD / PLAY			
Vision/Eyes	Blank & inattentive. Dark circles or sunken eyes. Dull, listless, eyes.	Clear, bright, curious eyes. Alert, and attentive. Easily scans and locates things.	Focus that excludes all else. Can't locate things in plain sight. Easily visually distracted.
Tendon & Joint Flexibility	Frequent strains and sprains. Unable to sit still.	Smooth, coordinated, pain-free movements in all joints.	Constant need for movement. Limited movement.
Anger	Rarely express anger or frustration even when being hurt or abused.	Can get mad, express feelings, and recover quickly.	Often angry or frustrated. Hurts others or destroys things. Holds grudges.
Play & Stress Relief	Avoid unpredictable activities. No time for pleasurable activities. Difficulty making decisions.	Spend daily time outdoors. Accept unpredictable events. Make decisions easily.	Crave new experiences & risks. Avoid schedules & rules. Difficulty changing perspective.
WATER / SLEEP			
Hearing	Unable to hear or understand. Miss information or directions.	Enjoy music, sounds. Hear and understand most spoken information & directions.	Sound sensitive. Extreme reactions to sounds.
Bones, Teeth, Resilience	Catch colds easily or suffer from seasonal allergies. Broken bones. Dental issues.	Rarely experience pain from joints, bones, or teeth. Few colds or allergies.	Chronic or severe joint, bone, or tooth pain. Colds & allergies that linger.
Fear	Fearless exploring the environment, new people or events. Take great risks.	Curious and confident exploring the environment. Not easily frightened by the unfamiliar.	Hesitant to explore the environment or stray from familiar surroundings and people.
Sleep & Imagination	Difficulty sleeping - less than 6 hours sleep/night. Wake often during night. Absence of dreams. Lack of imagination or creativity.	Fall asleep easily. Get 7-9 hours of sleep/day including naps. Dreams inspire creativity.	Sleeping more than usual or sleep during the day for long periods. Troubled by nightmares. Live mostly in imagination.

Worksheet 1.2: Healing Compass Clues Checklist *(continued)*

	Behaviors *Healing Approach*	Deficient / Erratic *Nurture / Soothe*	What We Want to See *Harmony & Balance*	Excess / Stuck *Channel / Motivate*
EARTH / EAT	Touch	Avoid or oblivious to textures and touch. Unaware of personal comfort for self or others.	Enjoy experiencing the world through texture and touch. Choose comfortable surroundings.	Continuous craving for physical comfort. Choose discomfort or even painful experiences.
	Muscle Strength & Endurance	Weakness and endurance limit activities. Frequently bump into objects or people.	Adequate strength, coordination, and endurance to engage in activities throughout the day.	Fitness, strengthening, and endurance activities edge out other interests and people.
	Anxiety or Overthinking	Rarely think or plan ahead. Often surprised by logical outcomes to choices.	Methodical. Consider options. Plan ahead. Trust in favorable outcomes.	Need to follow a plan to the letter. Obsession with perfection may halt completion of tasks.
	Mealtimes & Eating	Eat alone or erratically. Eat all day long. Crave sweets.	Enjoy sharing food with others. Confident in food choices and availability.	Mealtimes compromised by limited choices. Binging, purging, or eating very little.
METAL / WORK	Smell	Oblivious to smell. Unable to identify familiar smells.	Enjoy exploring the world smells. Can identify things by smell.	Super-sensitive to smells. Extreme reactions to smells.
	Skin Integrity & Coordination	Frequent bruises, cuts, rashes, sweating or dry skin. Need lots of repetitive practice to learn new skills.	Skin moist, clear, and free of cuts, bruises, rashes. Learn new movement skills easily.	Thick skin or patches of skin that heal slowly. Resist learning new movements.
	Sadness	Rarely feel grief or cry even when sad things happen. When crying may become inconsolable.	Cry easily when sad things happen. Get over minor upsets easily.	Usually feel sad. Unable to let go of sad feelings.
	Elimination & Inspiration	Occasional constipation or diarrhea. Surroundings become cluttered or dirty at times.	Regular – 1 to 3 BMs per day. Easy movements. Uncluttered, neat and clean surroundings.	Troubled by frequent constipation or diarrhea. Cluttered, dirty surroundings affect breathing.
FIRE / LOVE	Taste	Cautious about new flavors and experiences. Oblivious to flavors.	Enthusiastically explore a variety of flavors and experiences.	Limited to only familiar flavors and brands. Subtle differences can cause adverse reactions.
	Cardiovascular Health	Endurance, blood pressure, and heart rate may run low. Too tired to engage with the world.	Endurance, blood pressure, and heart rate allow for easy engagement with the world.	Endurance, blood pressure, or heart rate run high. Need constant engagement with the world.
	Joyfulness	Often unhappy. Rarely laughs. Avoids excitement or contact with others.	Feel content and happy most of the time. Laugh often and easily.	Laughs inappropriately. Constant craving for excitement even when that involves risk or injury.
	Social Engagement	Rarely spend time with family or friends. Avoid social events and meeting new people.	Make friends easily. Spend time with family or friends daily. Seek out social events. Enjoy meeting new people.	Constantly craving company of others. Calendar full of social events. Manage social difficulties with silliness or constant chatter.

Remember, we are the sole subject of our own experimental study. Each chapter begins with a somewhat poetic definition of the natural element associated with that practice. The rest of the chapter will outline the neurosensory and musculoskeletal aspects associated with the tissues, senses, and organs that resonate energetically with that natural element. The end of the chapter will focus on how to develop a habit that can help you transform discomforts into healthier, happier days and nights.

Developing a habit takes somewhere between 21 to 45 days of practice, depending on which scientific study we consult. In the chapters that follow, you will find directions for "Trying it Out," "Learning More," plus the Practices of "Setting an Intention and Doing It" for a month, "Making it Your Own" and "Sharing It." Trust your intuition as it directs you how to proceed with each practice. Sustainable Health means following our own knowledge of our body and our life. Some practices we may only try for a few days; others may develop into passionate improvisation or even a mission to share that practice with those around us. Some will lead us to learn more and choose to follow another path.

Healing is in our hands. Follow these "very strict" rules for healing:

- Have fun on your journey!
- Imagine all the possibilities you can dream!
- Eat what you love and love what you eat!
- Learn to create breathing room!
- Make friends and share your joy!

Exercise 1.3: Try Building a Personal Healing Compass

To create a beautiful representation of the conscious universe we need to seek out a special place in our home. Look around and get a sense of the energy around you. Most of us already have a haphazard energy center, a place where we set down lottery tickets, receipts, found objects of interest, jewelry we love, and birthday or anniversary cards. Find that place in your home. Once we have decided on where, we can begin.

1. Clear a space at least the size of a dinner plate, or larger. Dust it, clean it and make it ready.

2. Take something special—jewelry, a knick-knack, or other object we love—to represent us. Place that object in the center of the space.

3. Determine the direction of North, South, East and West using a compass or by watching to see where the sun (or moon) rises and sets. The sun and moon always rise in the East and set in the West. Their exact spot of rising and setting may wobble a bit on the horizon during the seasons, but they always come up exactly opposite of where they went down, and vice versa.

4. Put your right hand where the sun rises and your left hand where the sun sets. If your arms do not cross you are facing North. If your arms do cross over, you are facing South.

5. Find a small wooden object to place in the East, in the direction the sun rises every day. Perhaps we have something special made of wood. Maybe a piece of driftwood collected at the beach, or a saved flower from a loved bouquet. Perhaps we would like to place a living plant in this direction. Don't overthink or agonize, a wooden toothpick will do. We can rearrange and change our personal compass any time we want.

6. Find a special rock, crystal, or well-used or well-loved metal tool like a pen or penknife to place in the West, in the direction where the sun sets every day.

7. Get a candle, or small battery powered light to place in the South. If we use a real candle, we must make sure to put it in a safe, sturdy container that will not tip over or allow the flame to get close to any flammable object. Pay special attention to what is above the candle. Never light a candle below a shelf in a bookcase or near curtains. Never leave a candle unattended.

8. Put a small vessel of water in the North. Choose a container we love, or one that looks beautiful. Fill it with water from the tap, or collect some from a body of water we love.

Now we have created a personal Healing Compass, an energetic compass and gateway to the universe. We can spend a few minutes every day considering our Healing Compass and its relationship to our personal and environmental geography. We can make whatever adjustments, additions or improvements reflect our observation of these elements and their relationships with each other and to us.

Exercise 1.4: Set an Intention for Healing

Setting an intention is more than simply making a wish. An intention has an outcome, or destination, in mind. We need to spend some time crafting the words of our intention to direct its energy where we want. Our intention gives us a destination, but we may not always have control over how we get there. Here are the steps I recommend for setting an intention for healing.

1. Visualize a desired outcome and be specific. Rather than state "I want to lose weight" or "I want to be healthy" visualize what we would love to do at an ideal weight or state of health—something we cannot do right now. When we make requests of a conscious universe we may not have control over how we reach that end. "I want to lose 20 pounds" sounds very specific but any number of serious illnesses may result in extreme weight loss, without giving us the power to do those activities we most love to do.

2. State the desired outcome in a simple sentence that has no negative language. The conscious universe works simply in what many people refer to as a child's or angel's mind. "I don't want to get dementia" becomes "I want to get dementia" when we remove negative language. "I want to beat my grandchildren at Scrabble" or "I want to enjoy reading the classics my whole life" puts a powerful spin on the intention. "My whole life" doesn't set a date for either dementia or death, so that type of intention leaves the result up to the conscious universe, the environment and our DNA whereas "until I'm well into my 80s" could include getting dementia at 85 and living with it another decade or two.

3. Spend some time thinking about the power of words as we write down our intention. Put it on a piece of paper and place it at the center of our personal Healing Compass or post it on a mirror where we can have a daily reminder that we have given our body, mind, and spirit a mission of healing. As we go through each chapter we will be setting intentions that harness the elements associated with different aspects of healing.

CHAPTER 2

Wood Energies

Have Fun and Play

Stress: The confusion created when one's mind overrides the body's basic desire to choke the living daylights out of some jerk who desperately deserves it.

—Anonymous

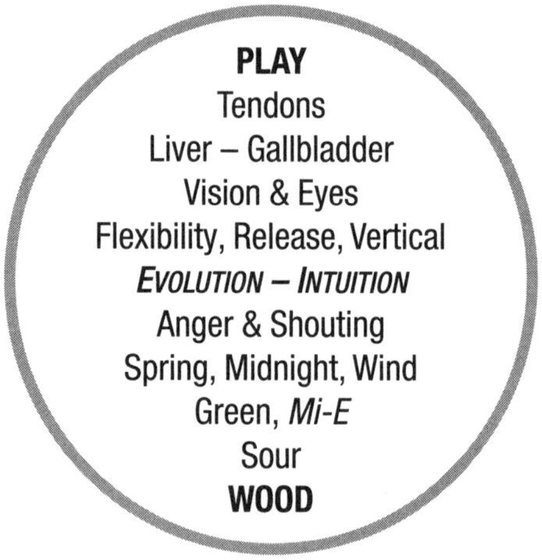

PLANTS GIVE US life—the air we breathe, food, shelter, clothing, and medicine. They commune with the plants around them via a fungal network in the earth and through taste and smell from wind and water. Plants entertain and support birds, bees, butterflies, poets, and artists. Lightning strikes the tallest trees, hurricanes topple even giant ones, and tornadoes drive straw deep into thick, protective bark. All manner of insects, birds, and animals nibble leaves, burrow into trunks, eat fruits, and carry trees' offspring far away to deposit them willy-nilly with a bit of fertilizer and a chance to settle new ground. Humans cultivate new species and mow down thousand-year-old forest communities, destroying tree species that may never reestablish themselves or recover lost relationships.

Most of us consider plants only in terms of how they affect us personally, yet plants know the deep connection of community on a cellular level. Flowers laugh, and leaves whisper. Plants endure, grow, and persist in the face of

PLAY
Tendons
Liver – Gallbladder
Vision & Eyes
Flexibility, Release, Vertical
EVOLUTION – INTUITION
Anger & Shouting
Spring, Midnight, Wind
Green, *Mi-E*
Sour
WOOD

Figure 2.1 Life Aspects Associated with Wood Energies

adversity. Every day they eat sunshine, make sugar, push through concrete, and dance with the wind. Lightning, tornadoes, hurricanes, and power saws—nothing completely stops plants. They creep over buildings and bury whole human civilizations, incautiously throwing their seeds to the wind and sending nutrients to fallen friends by keeping stumps alive for years (Wohlleben, 2016).

The plants we know first saw the light of day about 500 million years ago. We think of them as stationary, but they are constantly on the move—reaching out with roots, buds, and tendrils, sending their seeds all over the planet and floating on ocean currents.

Plants have a lot to teach us about letting go and smiling into the face of an ill wind.

Exercise 2.1: Make a Conscious Connection to Wood Energy

Go outside and take a look at what's growing there. Weeds come through concrete. Ivy covers walls. Bushes sprawl. Trees grow tall. Smell the roses. Breathe in the oxygenated air produced by plants. Think of some stories about the power of plants, like "Jack and the Beanstalk". Do you have any beloved plants or trees in your life?

Practice: Watch the Wind Blow and Playfully Let Go of Stress

Our practice for letting go of stress involves playfully interacting with trees, flowers, leaves, and the wind that moves through them. This eyes-wide-open meditation connects us to a conscious universe and brings us out of our own self-centered problems to a space where we can release stress, soak up sunshine, and shout into the wind.

Our busy, stress-filled lives release a host of hormones that drive emotions and actions we sometimes live to regret. Reconnecting with nature through observing living plants has proven power to soothe our moods and help us think more clearly (Craig, Logan, & Prescott, 2016).

Day by day, this practice strengthens our connection to the natural world and our resilience to stress. It provides us with the means to access a state of alertness and clarity, connection and confidence. Watch health and resilience improve as we reduce the inflammatory effects of stress.

Meditation, Contemplation, Prayer, and Daydreaming— What's the Difference?

Every group or tradition has a different way of making a connection with the divine or conscious universe.

Meditation usually involves focusing thoughts.

- Transcendental Meditation uses a mantra, a word, or sequence of syllables
- Zen meditation involves emptying the mind of all thought
- Guided meditation involves listening to words that will trigger imagination. We can write and record our own words or follow a prerecorded meditation created by someone else
- Moving meditation—walking, running, swimming, yoga, Tai Chi, or other actions that involve focused thought can serve as a form of meditation when they lead to a quiet mind

Contemplation involves focusing on a relationship with the divine. This closely resembles the practice described in this chapter. Teresa of Avila and John of the Cross detailed the Christian practice of contemplation in their 16th-century writings.

Prayer uses words for focus. These may be rote and repetitive or extemporaneous, heartfelt emotional silent or out loud conversations with the divine.

All of these practices eventually lead to a silent, peaceful space. When experienced practitioners permit scientists to connect them to machines that measure bodily functions, the scientists find that heart rate and respiration slow down and brain waves change. Many studies find that positive health outcomes result from a regular, daily meditation, contemplation, or prayer practice. Chapter Five will describe these changes in more detail.

People disagree about the benefits of daydreaming and whether it is another form of meditation. Watching the wind blow might seem something like daydreaming to you. If you can let yourself relax and your thoughts wander while watching the wind blow, consider it a form of meditation.

Stress: What Happens in the Body

Over millions of years, our bodies have developed and fine-tuned multiple ways of responding to stress through a complex web of interconnected neurons, hormones, and behaviors that enable us to survive both minor irritations and horrific circumstances. We come into the world with a fully functional sensory and autonomic nervous system that enables us to respond to and learn from our environment. At birth this system allows us to nurse by regulating our ability to suck, swallow, breathe, and vocalize. To do this we need to coordinate both conscious, and therefore voluntary, striated muscles that move our faces, tongues, and vocal chords with our unconscious, and involuntary, smooth muscles that control heart rate, breathing, and digestion (Porges, 2011).

As infants mature, these systems grow and optimize neural connections to include blinking, observation and imitation of facial expressions, and differentiation of human voices from background sounds. All of these neural connections enable increasingly complex social interactions. The complexity of our reactions to our surroundings, based on learning and experience, continues to develop as we go through life (Porges, 2011).

For decades, we thought of the autonomic nervous system as a binary system made up of a sympathetic system that enabled us to fight or flee, and a parasympathetic system that enabled us to calm ourselves for sleep, digestion, and similar "vegetative" processes. In the quest for "hard" science, neurobiologists largely ignored social relationships or words like kindness and compassion.

That has changed radically in the last few decades. Stephen Porges and Daniel Siegel, pioneers in interpersonal neurobiology, began to revise our understanding of human and mammalian nervous systems to accommodate increasing evidence that social bonds and communication form the core of what happens in our brains and bodies. Other biologists began looking more closely at other vertebrates, plants, and even microorganisms with this new notion of directed, or conscious, interaction. The connections between stress and our immune responses have proliferated from the work of many scientists.

After decades of observation and research with premature and full-term infants, Stephen Porges wrote *The Polyvagal Theory: Neurophysiological Foundations of Emotions, Attachment, Communication, and Self-Regulation,* which addresses how the vagus nerve acts as a conduit for integrating these responses between the brain and body.

Our vagus nerve is one of 12 pairs of nerves that leave our skull to reach various essential body structures. All of these cranial nerves play a part in sensing our environment, through nose, eyes, ears, tongue, and face, or move important muscles that facilitate sensation and our ability to engage with the environment for nourishment and social interaction. The rest of our nerves travel through our spinal cord before going out to tendons, joints, bones, muscles, skin, and other body tissues. All of our nerves bring back information about the environment and send out information about how to respond to it.

The vagus nerve travels to every organ in our body. About 80% of the vagus nerve brings information into the brain, and the rest takes information from the brain to individual organs, helping us regulate organ function and inflammatory responses to internal and external stress. Most of the vagus nerve transmits information relatively slowly, at a rate of 0.5 to 10 meters per second through unmyelinated axons. In mammals, myelin, a specialized fatty cell, coats about 20% of

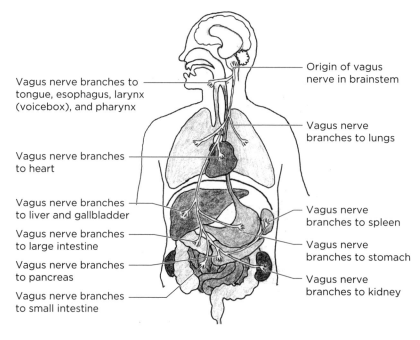

Vagus nerve branches to tongue, esophagus, larynx (voicebox), and pharynx

Origin of vagus nerve in brainstem

Vagus nerve branches to lungs

Vagus nerve branches to heart

Vagus nerve branches to liver and gallbladder

Vagus nerve branches to spleen

Vagus nerve branches to large intestine

Vagus nerve branches to stomach

Vagus nerve branches to pancreas

Vagus nerve branches to kidney

Vagus nerve branches to small intestine

Figure 2.2 Vagus nerve and its connection to the organs. 80% of this nerve brings information to the brain from all of the organs.

the axons in the vagus nerve and enables information to travel 10 times faster. As yet, this does not seem true for other classes of vertebrates, like reptiles and birds.

According to Porges, the vagus nerve, as well as the rest of the autonomic nervous system, has a primary goal of promoting *health, growth, and restoration*. He theorizes that in addition to fight-or-flight responses, the vagus nerve directs both a more primitive freeze-and-collapse response, as well as a "vagal brake" that interrupts these defensive responses, enabling social interactions essential for nursing in infants, as well as intimacy and social cooperation in older children and adults. The evolution of the myelinated vagal brake in mammals has made these social relationships possible (Porges, 2011).

Daniel Siegel's many publications, including *Mind: A Journey to the Heart of Being Human,* focus on the interaction of mind, brain, and relationships, through understanding the evolution of communication between the brain stem, limbic system, and cortex. The vagus nerve originates in the oldest part of our brain, the brain stem, also known as the "reptilian brain." The brainstem, together with the cerebellum, controls heart rate, breathing, body temperature, and balance. The brain stem communicates with the limbic system and cortex, integrating and regulating the above-mentioned physiological functions with more complex responses. The lim-

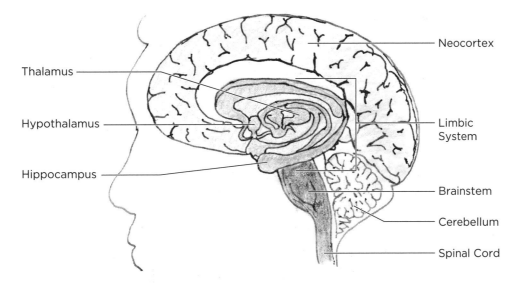

Figure 2.3   The brainstem, limbic system, and cortex of the brain. Our brainstem, also called the "reptilian brain" regulates essential life functions such as breathing, heart-rate, and digestion. It also primes us for fight, flight, and freeze responses. The limbic system mediates between our brainstem and cortex so that we can assess threats and override our more primitive fight, flight, and freeze responses by engaging socially.

bic system, often called our "mammalian" brain, regulates such complex responses as motivation, memory, emotion, and metabolism. Our primate cortexes, the familiar corrugated brain tissue that covers these older structures, governs even more complex integration, enabling reflection, relationships, and resilience.

Our responses to stress cover a wide-ranging and exceedingly complex network of neurons, neurotransmitters, hormones, metabolic functions, and behaviors. Science has opened many windows for understanding this process, and certainly we have much more to learn. What follows is a simplified version of five possible responses to threats.

1. *A threat to life caused by potentially fatal assaults or accidents will activate our most primitive response to freeze or even collapse.* When assaulted or severely injured, humans go into shock, dissociate, faint, feel paralyzed, or appear almost dead. These primitive, protective brain stem responses often ensure immediate survival. These types of responses reduce heart rate, respiration, body temperature, and other metabolic processes to conserve energy, confuse an enemy into overlooking us, or reduce effects (such as excessive bleeding) from a wound. In mammals, this kind of response works for short periods of time.

   Reptiles and amphibians developed this strategy to great advantage. When temperatures drop or life-giving water evaporates, these creatures can seek shelter and reduce their heart rates, respiration, and other metabolic processes to almost zero; they can maintain this condition for months or even years. Some mammals hibernate for a few months in the winter or estivate for a few months in the summer, but rarely longer. Mammals sleep with somewhat lowered heart rate and respiration during hibernation and estivation. Humans can sleep for long stretches when temperatures drop or food becomes scarce, therefore conserving energy and resources, but generally not for more than a few days at a time.

   Generally speaking, humans rely on a community of other people to recover from life-threatening assaults and accidents that cause a freeze or collapse response. Most research on this response has occurred anecdotally after the fact, when survivors relate their stories, especially those who have survived rape, assault, or warfare. Post-traumatic stress disorder (PTSD) will produce similar symptoms, triggered by body memories (limbic responses). These include: feeling cold, frozen, numb, or stiff and heavy in some part of our body; pale skin; restricted breathing; holding our breath; variable heart rate from pounding to slowing down; or loss of bowel and bladder continence (Breuning, 2017).

2. *A less serious life-threatening situation with an option for escape triggers our fight-or-flight response.* Often, we have a few initial moments of freezing, which enable us to size up the situation and choose some combination of fight, flight, or social engagement. In all threatening circumstances the adrenal glands on our kidneys begin releasing adrenaline and cortisol to prevent shock and dehydration. These hormones increase heart rate, respiration, blood sugar, memory, and vigilance. Blood leaves the digestive organs and flows toward muscles, preparing us for action. Sometimes vomiting empties a full stomach so we can move more easily.

   For the most part our neurohormonal response to this level of stress does not differentiate between fight or flight. We only see these differentiations in behavior. Fight responses include crying, muscle contractions, making fists, clenching jaws, glaring, low register threatening vocalizations, feelings of rage, and a desire to hurt or kill. Flight responses include tensed muscles; restless contractions in legs; wide, rapid eye movements to search for cover or an escape route; and movement (Breuning, 2017).

3. *Momentary stress caused by unfamiliar surroundings or surprising experiences engages the vagal brake.* Suppose you see a new face at work, friends organize a surprise party, or a family member raises or lowers their voice. These situations could trigger a fight, flight, or even a freeze response, and often do so for people with post-traumatic stress disorders. Ideally, this level of stress engages our myelinated vagal brake. We check in with higher cortical levels, engage our vision to assess others' facial features for signs of threat or aggression, and attend our hearing for high alerting shrieks or low threatening growls. We check our memories for past experiences with similar details and make the decision: engage with what we perceive as potentially enjoyable, recruit a fight-or-flight response, or completely freeze and collapse. We choose these three options in that order, using our most sophisticated cortical response first, and working our way down through the limbic system to a brain stem response if needed. All this occurs in a matter of seconds or less (Breuning, 2017).

4. *The vagal brake enables us to adopt another response to a threat,*

fawning. Fawning means just what it sounds like: Bambi, submitting to an aggressor in the absolutely cutest way possible. Suppose someone stronger or more socially powerful threatens us. We often identify these threats as bullying. We may fear that a fight response will result in defeat, possible injury, or even death. A flight response may involve leaving the protection of a larger group where we receive benefits we don't want to lose, our job, our family, our friends, or even an educational, religious, or professional institution. In those instances we may employ our vagal brakes to appease a bully, knowing we will live to fight back another day or another way (Breuning, 2017).

As I write this, the news is filled with stories, primarily from women, who have done just that. They accepted bullying behavior until their social power, both individually and collectively, enabled them to defeat those who had bullied them.

In many of these cases, years or even decades go by while younger, less powerful individuals acquire experience, status, and a group of supporters. Meanwhile, the bully ages, loses vigilance due to complacency, and offends or injures an ever-growing number of people who bide their time to strike back. History is replete with such stories about all kinds of bullies, from emperors to CEOs.

We see fawning in many mammalian species who live collectively. We like to think of humans as the apex of evolutionary development, so sometimes it comes as a shock to realize we behave much like our fellow mammals. However, knowledge does give us power to understand this response and give ourselves permission to use it wisely: forgiving ourselves and others for what we may perceive as past weakness, and exercising our power when we see an opportunity for success.

Hopefully, we have developed a vast repertoire of experiences that allow us to reflect back on positive relationships so that we have the kinds of resiliency we need to explore and learn from our environment. We develop these experiences in what Stephen Porges calls "co-regulation" (Porges, 2011). We set the stage for co-regulation during feedings in infancy. Infants must engage their vagal brake in order to integrate responses of sucking, swallowing, and breathing. Adult caregivers must engage their vagal brake to cuddle, coo to, and feed helpless newborn infants. Warmth through close contact (preferably skin to skin) and the calming sensations of feeding and eliminating build a foundation for co-regulation.

Infants grow lots of myelin in their brains during the first few months of life. As it grows, we begin to see that babies meet our gaze and soothe to cooing sounds. Then we engage in games like peek-a-boo and other playful interactions that elicit a mild threat followed by an immediately pleasurable calming, cuddling response. Other surprises happen, and infants learn to recognize consistency in the environment and, hopefully, a sense of security that their needs will be met. Communications between members of the family and community become increasingly complex, memories multiply, and the child develops resilience based on these relationships and the ability to reflect on them in novel situations.

5. *Continuous low-level threats employ the vagal brake to engage in fawning, which may provide momentary relief, while keeping our cortisol and adrenaline high enough to maintain vigilance against another threat.* When the situation, or our memories of similar situations, engages a fawning response, we may continue to secrete sufficient stress hormones to raise blood glucose, increase our heart rate, and activate other inflammatory responses that contribute to inflammatory diseases affecting every organ along the vagal nerve. We find that groups who consistently face these types of daily threats to life have higher rates of stress hormones, such as salivary cortisol. Scientists generally understand that repeated exposures to these stress hormones makes people more susceptible to chronic diseases, such as cancer, heart disease, diabetes, and obesity, as well as addiction (Alexander, 2011).

Poverty; discrimination based on race, gender, disability, or age; and other inherent physical differences raise cortisol in the bloodstream. People who face these kinds of daily threats to life—lack of food, shelter, and security—also have higher rates of chronic diseases, such as diabetes, heart disease, and obesity, relative to those with higher social status who feel secure in their access to food, shelter, and security (Breuning, 2017).

Calming the Body After Stressful Experiences

Our bodies have developed a wide range of ways to reduce and reverse these biochemical responses to stress. Being prepared to defend and protect ourselves is important, but so are health, growth, and restoration. We need to be able to calm down quickly once a threat resolves. Our bodies have exquisite, multileveled, and redundant pathways to do so. Just as the autonomic system has ways to prepare us for self-defense and protection, it also has many pathways to restore us to a state where we can heal and grow.

1. *Eating not only soothes anxiety, it restores nutrients lost during responses to a stressful and threatening situation.* The foods our body directs us to eat after stress are sugars and fats—our "comfort foods." These restore energy lost during fight, flight, freeze, and fawn responses. The cortisol released during periods of threats and stress causes us to store the excess triglycerides these foods produce in and around our organs (visceral fat). This makes sense, because it provides a layer of protective padding we can readily metabolize. More frequent fasting than feasting, or a high ratio of muscle to fat, will rev up our metabolism and help us burn all kinds of fat, beginning with visceral fat. When an excess of visceral fat stays with us, it leads to insulin resistance and metabolic disorders, such as diabetes and heart disease (Lustig, 2013).

   Frequent secretion of cortisol kills neurons that regulate food intake, so continuous, low-level stress contributes to obesity. Unfortunately, studies show that food restraint from dieting (usually done in the service of weight loss) also seems to cause effects similar to other kinds of chronic stressors—like the poverty, discrimination, and environmental insecurity mentioned above (Lustig, 2013).

   In immediate fight-or-flight situations, cortisol has a well-defined feedback loop in the brain that causes the hypothalamus to shut down its production. That doesn't seem to happen with chronic stress. Memories of trauma or constant states of vigilance cause the kinds of cortisol responses that lead to overeating comfort foods and all that entails.

2. *Stimulation of pleasure, or hedonic, pathways in the brain releases "happy hormones" like dopamine, serotonin, and endorphins, which make us feel*

good, at least for a while. Eating triggers these hedonic pathways. So do movement, play, and most of the drugs involved in addiction. Each of these happy hormones acts on the brain in a different way.

Dopamine gets us focused on what we want and keeps us focused until we get it. Then it stops flowing, and we have to look for something else that we want, or a larger quantity of the same thing we just got (Breuning, 2017).

Serotonin helps us maintain our social position. When we have a higher status in a group we get more benefits, chiefly first access to food and fawning versus aggressive responses from other group members. Studies show that those with high status have lower cortisol in their saliva. We need almost constant stimulation to keep serotonin flowing, which can lead to constant needs for recognition or dominance (Breuning, 2017).

Endorphins, often called the body's opiates, help us mask pain with a feeling of euphoria. Endorphins start to flow only after injury and last for about 20 minutes. Self-injurious behaviors and lots of pharmaceuticals (both legal and not) mimic or stimulate the release of these hormones (Breuning, 2017).

All of our stress and happy hormones operate in bursts rather than continuously. Dopamine, serotonin, and endorphins get triggered by events and then quickly dissipate. Overeating, taking drugs, and indulging in addictive behaviors have inherent problems that can lead to mental and physical disability, especially when employed to relieve chronic, daily stresses. Fortunately, we have another way to reset our biochemistry.

3. *Playful interactions that build relationships release another happy hormone, oxytocin.* Oxytocin gets triggered by being close to those we trust, preferably close enough to touch. Those bursts stop when we feel separated and alone. We get oxytocin bursts when in relationships with people and other animals we trust (Breuning, 2017).

Oxytocin levels rise considerably during nursing, childbirth, and love-making, but smaller bursts happen in any trusting and pleasurable interchange, including those with our pets. To get these kinds of bursts, we must use our vagal brake to override our older evolutionary drives to fight, flee, or freeze. Stephen Porges calls the way we co-regulate in a relationship with a trusted companion, something all mammals must learn to do— *play.* Oxytocin has enabled us to improve our survival odds in cooperative groups. Most of us gain expertise with this hormone in childhood games where we learn to make rules, break rules, and go along to get along.

Play and Mentally Letting Go of Stress

Whenever we experience stress hormones, our minds immediately fabricate a story about our response. For the most part this helps us remember how to behave in similar stressful situations, but sometimes the story comes out of an earlier stressful situation and not our current circumstances.

We all know someone who seems happy in spite of economic setbacks, separation from loved ones, or serious illness. How do they do it?

Martin Seligman, Mihaly Csikszentmihalyi, and other psychologists who studied happiness developed the field of positive psychology. They agree that these people can see their lives from a different perspective. Quite simply, they change beliefs by telling themselves another story.

Beliefs create thoughts.
Thoughts create emotions.
Emotions create actions.
Actions create health.

If we *believe* that things never work out our way, we may *think* the world is out to get us. We get *angry* at what we perceive as the cause of our bad luck. With cortisol flowing, we can use freeze, fight, flee, and fawn, strategies that proved successful in the past, but don't always work for us in our present circumstances. These might include behaviors like giving up and spending all day in front of the TV, arguing about almost everything, moving out, or making nice with the bullies.

If we *believe* that life, like any game, provides spectacular opportunities for learning and loving, we can begin to *imagine* lots of ways to engage. If we generally *enjoy* playing, we *celebrate* our wins and *shrug off* our losses. Cortisol, adrenaline, and the happy hormones live in harmony and balance through flexibility in the ways we perceive and tell our stories. Disaster might lead to new opportunities. Pain could result in lessons learned. Survival against all odds may well grow an unshakable faith in the future.

How do these happy people change their story? Positive psychologists tell us genetics plays a part, as does experience. Happy people have practiced retelling their story to themselves and others. Happy people feel emotions deeply and then let them go, in bursts that flow like their neurotransmitters—cortisol, adrenaline, and the happy hormones. They don't forget. In fact, they remember what signs let them know a threat is imminent; how to react for survival; and, *most importantly,* how to let all those stresses go afterwards. The genetics side of this equation depends on luck at conception, but the experience side rests squarely within our powers of learning through repetitive practice (Siegel, 2016). We will go into this more deeply in Chapter 5.

We develop resilience and learn to let go of stress by playing with danger. As infants, survival depends on being in the arms of a caring adult. Everything else brings with it a threat to survival. Infants learn to play with danger when adults make scary faces or silly noises and then laugh (peek-a-boo). As soon as children can point, gurgle, and pull away, they begin playing with relationships: who looks and listens (safe), and who doesn't (unsafe). Soon they begin playing with gravity and its effects on their own bodies and the objects they launch—or have launched at them. They observe what older children and adults do and imitate those behaviors. Cuts and bruises abound, but injuries heal, providing varying amounts of endorphin and dopamine, teaching us our physical limits. We learn social and emotional limits by which behaviors get praised (resulting in serotonin and oxytocin bursts) and which produce threats, warnings, or punishment (stimulating cortisol and adrenaline bursts). We develop persistence when we decide we want to do something difficult and succeed (for a burst of dopamine). The older we get, the more complicated and interconnected these responses get.

The experiences we have as young children, and those we have at puberty build our strongest neural pathways. During these stages our bodies grow more myelin to make rapid neural connections. Sometimes something bad, like physical or sexual abuse, will set off bursts of cortisol and adrenaline. But what if that threatening situation gets paired with something that triggers a burst of happy hormones like candy and dopamine, special attention and serotonin, drug use and endorphins, or affection and oxytocin?

Doing something antisocial, which generally triggers an unpleasant oxytocin deficit, might get paired with happy hormones such as getting what we want and dopamine, exerting power over others and serotonin, self-injury and drug use with endorphins, or sexual release and oxytocin. We get bursts of these happy hormones in spite of the potentially negative social-emotional costs of separation and isolation that reduce the release of oxytocin.

Every life usually has a wide range of happy, sad, scary, painful, and worrisome experiences. When "good" things happen we learn how to repeat them. When "bad" things result in successful survival we learn important lessons. When bad things result in continued suffering, we learn survival approaches that don't always help us out later on in life.

Adults who grew up in abusive situations as children or adolescents often react with fight, flight, freeze, and fawn responses when something about their present environment triggers a memory from the past. These responses cause our bodies to release stress hormones. When we feel safe and surrounded by friends, we can employ our vagal brakes to set off happy hormones through playful engagement. We all have many opportunities to trigger our happy hormones. Reaching a goal, even a small one like checking a box on our "to do" list, releases dopamine. Successfully exercising our rights and sticking up for ourselves releases serotonin. Enduring discomfort or pain to help others releases both endorphins and oxytocin (Breuning, 2017).

Play keeps our hormones moving when survival stakes are low. We usually don't worry about getting hurt or killed during play times, so we won't produce the same levels of cortisol and adrenaline as a high-stakes, threatening situation would. Games produce enough cortisol and adrenaline to get us interested and engaged, and plenty of opportunities to set off the happy hormones. Games also give us practice engaging our vagal brakes, especially when we play at being an aggressor. Unless we exercise restraint in games like tag, wrestling, and the like, our playmates will soon leave us for more pleasurable experiences.

In his book, *Free to Learn: Why Unleashing the Instinct to Play Will Make Our Children Happier, More Self-Reliant, and Better Students for Life,* psychologist Peter Gray points out that children in unstructured play rarely sustain the types of injuries involved in organized sports such as Little League. As soon as we start to worry about outcomes, play becomes something else— work or punishment.

Having fun and enjoying what we're doing, the people we're with, and the world around us keeps our happy hormones flowing. We can enjoy winning for a burst of dopamine; praise and admiration for a burst of serotonin; or exercising our vagal brake to stay positively engaged with our playmates after losing, for bursts of oxytocin. Weight lifting, running, and other endurance sports usu-ally involve some relatively minor trauma to muscles that activates endorphins, producing the athlete's "high." However, when done to extreme, these forms of play can lead to repetitive motion injuries, or even more serious trauma.

All mammals play. Young mammals learn how to develop physical skills, solve problems, and get along with others from their games. Adult mammals play to maintain relationships and discharge stress. Play keeps our bodies fit, our minds active, our social relationships flexible, and our spirits high.

In December 1914, Ernest Shackleton led a trans-Antarctic expedition. About six weeks into this journey, his ship, the *Endurance*, got stranded in pack ice on the Weddell Sea. In the nine months that followed he ordered his crew to play games and perform skits to keep themselves alert and ready to con-tinue their journey as soon as the ice broke in spring. Unfortunately, the mov-ing pack ice crushed their ship. Shackleton and the crew continued on with a grueling and harrowing journey of endurance and resilience that eventually resulted in Shackleton's rescue of his entire crew on August, 30, 1916 (Lansing, 2014). Their story stands as one of heroic reflection, relationship, and resil-ience under unimaginable stress, and their nine months of playful interaction while stranded at the start of that journey surely set the stage for their later successful survival.

Exercise 2.2: Egging on Anger

Take an egg and go outside to a place that has some trees. Think about a recent incident that stimulated a flight, fight, or fawning response. Imagine that story taking place as an entire play within the egg. Who did what? Give emotions free-rein. Pile on the blame. Get completely self-righteously angry. Imagine revenge scenarios. Put them all there inside that egg.

Then with a mighty shout hurl the egg at the nearest tree. Our anger in all of its glory has just become an offering to the tree spirits (birds and other crea-tures who like to eat eggs).

Now that anger is gone, we can tell ourselves a new story. We can re-imagine the incident from a new perspective, one that gives us plenty of oxytocin, dopa-mine, and serotonin. Change the storyline to an outcome full of connection, success, and recognition. Focus on our own positive outcome, rather than what happens to the other characters. This may take a lot of imagination! Remember it's our story and we can write any happy ending we want. Look around and find a plant or a bird to help you remember this new scenario. Take a twig, leaf, or feather from your plant or bird ally as a reminder that you have the power to change perspective. Place that token in the east and use it when you need supportive Wood energy to manage stress.

How Did "Play" Become a Four-Letter Word?

Play keeps us healthy, and most of us don't get enough of it.

Ethologists, scientists who study animal behavior, define "play" as any voluntary, enjoyable activity that does not lead directly to survival behaviors such as getting food or offspring. They have documented these behaviors in mammals, fish, reptiles, and birds (Burghardt, 2015; Emory & Clayton, 2015). This definition of play encompasses scrolling on cell phones and computers, as well as drawing in the dirt, daydreaming, reading for pleasure, and playing poker. Why is play so important that not only mammals but a whole host of other vertebrates do it?

It appears that play keeps us regulated and able to devote ourselves to growth, health, and restoration so that, when necessary, we have the strength, flexibility, and stamina to use fight, flight, freeze, and fawn responses for survival. We mammals use our vagal brakes to foster the cooperative behaviors that give us time to raise our young and teach them how to skillfully employ their natural, genetic, and intuitive talents.

Somewhere along the road from living in small bands with only the tools we could carry, play evolved from an integral part of everyday life to a rare and coveted event. Instead of forming the centerpiece of daily life, play happened only during those odd moments not consumed by often less than pleasant, productive work.

Marshall Sahlins, author of *Stone Age Economics*, and other anthropologists have documented that indigenous cultures in their original environments (as opposed to those relocated to make way for industrial progress) spend only 3 to 5 hours a day in pursuit of food, clothing, and shelter. This leaves them with a lot of time to pursue what we might describe as recreational and creative pursuits—or play.

Medieval peasants, who worked from sunup to sundown during spring, summer, and harvest, then considerably less time during winter, by custom observed a day of rest weekly, on Sunday, as well as 150 partial or full "holy days of obligation" that required eschewing work to attend religious celebrations, church services, processions, and dramatic plays (Eisenstein, 2011). This amounts to more than every other day off. Work involved much physical labor, and peasants endured a fair amount of discriminatory treatment, food insecurity, and strife, but they had a lot of time to do nothing. They had time for *healing, growth,* and *restoration.* They had time for *reflection.* They had time to socialize and grow *relationships.* They had time to develop *resilience.* They had time to play.

Sixteenth-century painter Pieter Bruegel left behind numerous examples of people playing, including his painting "Children's Games," in which we can identify children engaging in games still played by children in the 21st century. For the most part children learned all these games from other children, without any adult intervention, yet today if we go to a local school playground, public park, or vacant lot we might not see many of these games in progress.

We have reduced the amount of time allowed for play tremendously in the

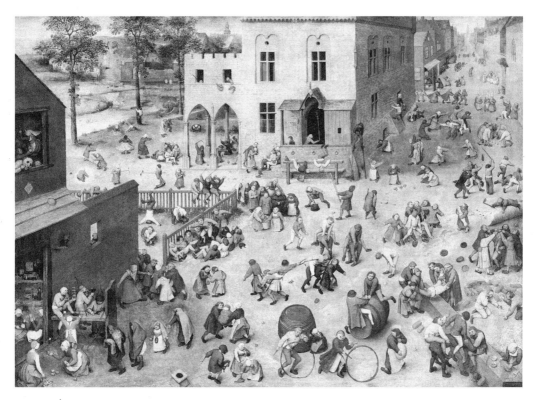

Figure 2.4 Children's Games by Pieter Bruegel. All around the courtyard children and some adults engage in a variety of games. Which ones can you recognize? Used with permission from KHM-Museumsverband.

last few decades, not just for adults, but for children as well. Doing so has led to chronic health problems from lack of exercise, as well as problems in mental health and learning. Many children's games have all but disappeared, and often their survival depends on adult teachers rather than a child-to-child lineage (Gray, 2013).

Psychologists have used the Minnesota Multiphasic Personality Inventory (MMPI) to assess mental health in college-age students since 1938. A version developed for adolescents has been given to high school students since 1950. Rates of anxiety and depression have risen steadily from those times to the present. During the same time span the amount of time children spend in unsupervised or lightly supervised play, such as school recess, has steadily declined (Gray, 2013). Richard Louv, author of *Last Child in the Woods,* has documented a similar decline in outdoor play and has identified a condition he calls "nature deficit disorder," which impacts both children and adults.

Nature deficit disorder has no official acceptance in medical literature, but Louv's use of this term and his accounts of adult and child experiences in nature have attracted a lot of attention from clinicians and educators. A number of studies have yielded results that show improvements in academic test scores, job productivity, and social relationships, plus reduced biochemical markers of stress, increased endorphins and dopamine, as well as other positive health benefits associated with spending time outdoors, in natural environments full of vegetation, open spaces, rivers, and streams (Louv, 2008).

Dopamine, our reward hormone, gets stimulated by substances such as alcohol, cocaine, and amphetamines, as well as comfort foods. These substances can trigger us to release endorphins that mask pain with euphoria (Olive, Koenig, Nannini, & Hodge, 2001). If we are experiencing physical or emotional pain, we want more euphoria to cope with it. This sets up a neurohormonal cycle of addiction. Relieving pain through other pathways enhances our abilities to cope, because it gives us a variety of options. Heat and cold, stretching, massage, and other manual therapies often help with tissue pain, but nothing seems to work better than play when it comes to alleviating emotional pain.

In 1978, psychologist Bruce Alexander conducted a series of experiments now known as the Rat Park experiments (Alexander, 2011). During the last half of the 20th century, academic and popular media supported a theory of addiction that proposed that anyone exposed to drugs of abuse such as heroin, morphine, and alcohol would become addicted. Much of this theory relied on experiments done on starved and isolated rats in bare cages equipped only with water, or water laced with the drug under investigation. These rats continuously consumed the drugs, often to point of death due to overdose. The results of this research made its way into public service announcements advising viewers that even a one-time use of these drugs would lead to potentially fatal addictions.

Alexander, aware that rats in nature live in highly social groups, wondered if part of the addictive process resulted from "solitary confinement," a condition known to create abnormal, self-injurious, and psychotic behaviors in humans and other primates. He and his colleagues at Simon Fraser University constructed a communal living space they nicknamed Rat Park, because it had lots of play equipment (wheels, cans, boxes, and wood shavings) as well as other rats of both sexes—and not long after starting the study, lots of rat pups.

After carrying out a variety of experiments with Rat Park, these researchers found that:

- Rats in Rat Park consumed much, much less morphine (almost 20 times less than rats in solitary cages).
- They consistently refused morphine water and preferred plain water.
- Rats isolated in cages and fed nothing but morphine water for 57 days chose plain water and voluntary withdrawal when moved to Rat Park.
- Nothing the researchers tried in Rat Park caused the rats living there to increase their consumption of morphine water. (Alexander, 2011)

Despite the lack of recognition these studies received in academic and addiction-treatment circles, Alexander went on to pursue this line of reasoning using historical accounts and interviews with people addicted to all kinds of things from drugs to gambling, shopping, and Internet use. He documents these findings and suggestions for the future in his book, *The Globalization of Addiction: A Study in Poverty of the Spirit.*

Although play might not be the answer to all our problems, making more time to play definitely reduces stress and helps us get the happy hormones flowing. Indeed, part of the success of 12-step programs to battle addictions probably reflects the supportive community they offer their members, which counteracts feelings of isolation.

Outdoor play and connecting with plants and nature have their own positive effects as well. Because our vagal nerve connects to all our organs, exercising it through play of various kinds has shown positive effects on health.

Shinrin-yoku, or "forest bathing" in English, has become an accepted health practice in Japan. Versions of *shinrin-yoku* have spread throughout Asia and even made their way across the Pacific to North America. Yoshifumi Miyazaki, medical doctor and professor at Chiba University, about 20 miles outside of Tokyo, pioneered *shinrin-yoku.* He has conducted many studies documenting the effects of aimlessly walking among trees and its capacity to lower stress-related indicators such as cortisol in saliva, heart rate, respiration, and blood pressure (Park, Kagawa, Kasetani, Tsunetsugu, & Miyazaki, 2009). He often collaborates with Qing Li, a professor at Nippon Medical School in Tokyo, on studies that show how forest bathing boosts our immune responses.

When plants eat sunshine via photosynthesis, they take in carbon dioxide and water to produce glucose. This process releases oxygen into the air. Whenever we surround ourselves with plants, we increase our available oxygen. We need that oxygen for our own metabolism of glucose and triglycerides into energy. Plants also emit phytoncides to protect themselves from germs and insects. Li's research indicates that being in the presence of trees and plants stimulates production of our own natural killer (NK) white blood cells, which boosts our immune system (Li, 2009).

Researchers from the World Health Organization's Regional Office for Europe used geographical mapping and health data to correlate the effects of living near parks, trees, and plants. The 2016 studies showed significantly better results for those who live near green spaces, and these results held true regardless of income, education, or employment, which also affect health outcomes.

Even simply viewing plants also speeds recovery after stressful events such as a math test or illness. A classic study done by Robert Ulrich in 1984 found that for a group of patients recovering from gallbladder surgery, those with a window that looked out onto trees had shorter postoperative hospital stays, less need of medication for pain, slightly lower scores on a measure of postsurgical complications, and fewer complaints from the nurses treating them (Ulrich, 1984).

Psychologists Rachel and Stephen Kaplan developed a theory called "attention restoration" based on studying their subjects' ability to improve concentration after spending time in nature or viewing scenes from nature. Other psychologists have pursued similar studies of how spending time in nature, or simply viewing natural scenery, improves attention as well other executive functions such as motivation, short-term memory, and organization. Their research has much promise for people struggling with attention deficit disorders and brain injuries that directly impact these executive functioning skills (Krisch, 2014).

Connecting to a Conscious Universe Through Plants

We often feel isolated and alone when separated from our friends and family. Our culture has denied our connections to other species on this amazing planet for close to 400 years. Isaac Newton ushered us into a world dominated by the mathematics of gravity and a view of the universe as a giant machine with only one sentient species, *homo sapiens*. Fifty years earlier, Galileo was sentenced to a decade of house arrest for suggesting that the Earth revolved around the sun and was not, as commonly believed, the center of the universe. He begged his accusers to simply take a look through his telescope, but they refused to do so.

Almost four centuries later, despite a multitude of scientific studies, we still cling to the notion of humans and human needs as all important—in effect, the center of the universe. We need to let go of this notion and the stressful struggle we have taken on in our attempts to control both nature and the much larger universe.

We can learn a lot about flexibility and "going with the flow" from trees and plants. They have 500 million years of DNA wisdom to our paltry 3 million. We humans are simply one very busy and often destructive species on a planet full of an almost unimaginable diversity of sentient beings—beings with consciousness. Once we establish a relationship to these other beings, we no longer need to feel alone. Of course, to do so we need to learn which beings and which circumstances lead to safety (most of them) and which ones might require us to fight, flee, freeze, or fawn (some of them, especially other humans!).

Peter Wohlleben introduces us to the community of plants in his best-selling book, *The Hidden Life of Trees: What They Feel, How They Communicate*. Plants move very slowly compared to us. We can outrun all plants, save those in our imaginations. As long as we only eat those plants we know taste good and avoid those that make us itch when we touch them, we can consider plants as nurturing companions.

Can trees communicate? We all must decide that question for ourselves, but simply because we consider other beings nonsentient doesn't make them so. Botanists, who study how trees and plants sense the world around them, have found that plants certainly do feel and respond to all kinds of chemical and electrical signals. They follow the path of the sun and the rhythms of the moon and seasons. Wohlleben describes how trees in Africa change the flavor of their leaves to discourage giraffes from eating them. Then they warn the surrounding trees about the giraffes.

Mammal neurons transmit neuroelectric signals very quickly, measured in meters per second. Slow, unmyelinated nerves move at 0.5 to 2 meters per second. Myelinated nerves send impulses in ranges from 3 to 120 meters per second, depending on the type of nerve. Trees send electrical impulses at about one centimeter a second (Wohlleben, 2016), or 50 times slower than mammals' slowest nerves.

It takes a while for the tree to make its leaves less palatable, and longer still for the first tree to send messages through the complex interconnected root network of the soil to other trees. The speedy giraffes can leisurely munch on one tree until its leaves become too bitter and then gracefully take a few steps along to another tree who hasn't yet learned about the giraffe problem, to munch on more tasty leaves (Wohlleben, 2016). Giraffes eat fewer leaves per tree and spread the damage across a wider range of trees, and so the grove protects itself.

Best Houseplants for Air Filtration

Our air quality has deteriorated over the last few decades, especially in cities. Many people buy expensive and useful home air filtration systems. If we can't fit one of these into our budget, we can use house plants, which filter air and add oxygen for a fraction of the cost of an air filter. We can even explore around garden centers, rescue a discarded plant, revive it with water, and get our air filtered for free!

In 1989 NASA sponsored a white-paper report on using plants to filter air contaminants from enclosed spaces, preventing what they called "sick building" syndrome. They then tested twelve of these plants in their filtration system. [Read their report, "Interior Landscape Plants for Indoor Air Pollution Abatement," to see the simple filtration system they built (Wolverton, Johnson, & Bounds, 1989).]

All of the plants they tested improved air quality in sealed chambers tested over a two-year period. These plants cleared the air of the common toxic pollutants trichloroethylene, benzene, and formaldehyde. Probably most plants would do the same. A list of the plants they tested follows. The paper was cosponsored by the Associated Landscape Contractors of America, who presumably chose plants for hardiness indoors.

Bamboo palm, *Chamaedorea seifritzii*

Chinese evergreen, *Aglaonema modestum*

English ivy, *Hedera helix*

Ficus, *Ficus benjamina*

Gerbera daisy, *Gerbera jamesonii*

Janet Craig, *Dracaena deremensis "Janet Craig"*

Marginata, *Dracaena marginata*

Mass cane/Corn cane, *Dracaena massangeana*

Mother-in-law's tongue, *Sansevieria laurentii*

Peace lily, *Spathiphyllum "Mauna Loa"*

Pot mum, *Chrysanthemum morifolium*

Warneckei, *Dracaena deremensis "Warneckei"*

We can make our homes and workspaces both more beautiful and healthier with houseplants.

Flexibility and Flow: The Healing Power of Wood Energies

Figure 2.1 shows aspects of life that Five Element Theory associates with the Wood element. Plants demonstrate flexibility, an ability to grow and adapt to new situations. Flexibility of body manifests itself in our vision and our tendons. Flexibility of thought requires us to move around and see the world from different perspectives. Flexibility of emotion requires a well-developed vagal brake to make quick shifts between fun, fight, flight, freeze, and fawn responses. Flexibility also requires release of tension, ideas, and anger.

Our eyes use a variety of muscles and nerves to change their shape and the shape of the lenses within our eyes. This flexibility enables us to see things at extreme distances or close at hand. Maintaining our focus on an object at a fixed distance, like a book or computer screen, reduces our visual flexibility, as do glasses and other lenses even though they also provide much needed clarity for modern eyes. Good vision benefits from constant movement, focus, and release.

Tendons attach our muscles to bone or other tendons. They also work best when flexible. Tendons have small sensory organs, called Golgi tendon organs, embedded in them. Golgi tendon organs play a protective role in our use of muscle strength. If you have ever picked up a box or other object that was too heavy for you to easily manage and yet continued to carry it until you experienced a sudden loss of strength that caused you to drop that heavy weight, then you have benefited from the Golgi tendon organs' protective function. It signals the muscles to let go before they tear a tendon's attachment away from the bone (Greene & Roberts, 2017).

Tendons benefit from hydration and movement to maintain their flexibility. Brittle, unused tendons tear away from bone much more easily than supple tendons that retain their flexibility through good hydration and frequent stretching movements. Reaching and bending our spine and limbs in all directions keeps us flexible and ready to react at a moment's notice.

Of all the elements in the Healing Compass, only Wood can adapt and change. Wood grows upward, with most of its growth occurring in spring. Plants grow faster at night, and Wood energy governs the hours from 11 p.m. to 3 a.m., according to Five Element Theory. As we will see in the next chapter, sleeping during these hours provides the most benefit for health, growth, and restoration.

Of all the weather conditions possible, wind carries much danger for plants, who have developed a multitude of strategies for coping with damp, dry, heat, and cold. Trees can lose limbs, tops, and even their attachment to the earth in high winds. Trees also benefit from wind. They communicate through the wind

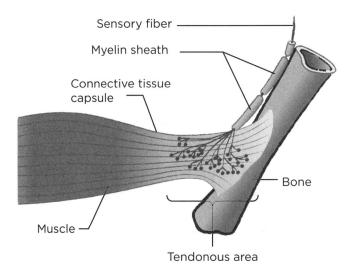

Figure 2.5 Golgi Tendon Organ. The small spray of nerves where the tendon attaches to bone causes the muscle to release its tension and let go when a force threatens to tear that attachment.

using aromatic chemicals, and they use it for movement, to carry their pollen and seeds.

Plants have flavors that include sweet nectars and fruits; sour fruits and leaves; bitter leaves, buds, and barks; as well as spicy and savory roots and barks. Some plants, like celery, even taste salty. Five Element Theory identifies sour as the flavor of Wood. For herbalists, understanding how these flavors correspond and interact based on Five Element Theory helps them choose which ones to use when treating a client (Ody, 2017).

Have Fun: Play with Life

Play keeps us flexible. It keeps us moving, using our eyes and our vagal brakes to keep our responses lively and ready for the never-ending variety of demands that life puts on us. Through the interaction of our hormones and our autonomic nervous system, stress often leads to anger and depression, which take a toll on our liver and gallbladder. Stress depletes the bile we secrete to digest fats and often leads to bloating as the day goes on and we accumulate more stress (Chida, Sudo, & Kubo, 2006).

Let go of stress with active play, tossing a ball around, or shouting into the wind. Run. Jump for joy. Climb a tree or some stairs for a change of perspective. Feel angry, then shout and throw things. Let anger go with tears or laughter. Anger causes us the most damage when we hold onto it. Let go of resentments.

Practice Having Fun! Watch the Wind Blow

This practice has us use our eyes as nature intended, looking for movement, shifting our focus, turning our heads to follow the path of a bird, a leaf drifting to the ground, or a cloud passing by. Doesn't that sound delightful?

Our eyes, the sensory organ associated with Wood frequencies, embody flexibility as constant adjustments of size and shape accommodate our focus to near and far while watching movement. Because most of us keep our focus on short-range reading and desk work, our eyes have become less flexible. The amount of enjoyable, nonrepetitive physical movement we do in a day has decreased and with it the flexibility of our tendons, which increases our risk for sprains and strains. Not surprisingly, we also seem to have lost flexibility in our emotions and in our ability to let go of anger, frustration, and stress.

This practice seems quite simple and easy at first glance. Even the idea of spending time watching the wind blow may sound soothing. Very quickly we come to realize that "doing nothing" triggers a deep-seated urge to get up and get busy. Sitting with this urge, breathing in and out, and focusing on watching movement helps us take a few moments of respite to let go of everyday worries and resentments.

Watching the wind blow is a form of meditation. Letting go of a busy mind challenges everyone who has ever meditated. Hundreds of books on meditation offer advice for getting through this stage, such as paying attention to breathing; holding postures of various kinds; and focusing on a light, a mantra, or a religious icon. All of them advise us to be gentle with ourselves, to recognize that loss of focus happens to everyone. The repetitive practice of acknowledging distracting thoughts and letting them go makes it get easier. Perfection doesn't seem to come to us in this life, but letting go of the need to reach perfection will set us free to enjoy each moment.

Meditation gives us release from a busy mind, release from resentments, and a chance to clear our neurohormonal slate to make room for new opportunities, fresh perspectives, and a sense of connection with the conscious universe. Doing this has wide-ranging positive effects on physical and mental health.

Exercise 2.3: Try Doing Nothing

Explore this practice by taking some time to sit outside, when weather and circumstance permit, or indoors looking out a window. When we can't find trees, we can look for movement of clouds, birds, people, vehicles, or even those ubiquitous plastic grocery bags caught in a breeze.

Become aware of movement, of life all around us. We do not live in a stationary world. Everything moves and changes constantly. Observe this flow.

Approach this practice with a sense of fun.

Grab a beverage if that strikes your fancy.

Remember being a kid with no commitments and no worries. We could stare out a window or up at the sky. We could watch ants scurry about their business. Eventually some grown-up would call us back to "attention." We're the grown-ups now, so we can tell that voice in our head to "buzz off!"

Watch a dog or cat. How do they sit so still, just watching? Copy them. Let them teach us how to watch for movement.

How long can we enjoy sitting still and playing with our eyes? What thoughts come up? Can we let them go?

Sometimes it takes a few minutes to see movement. If we give ourselves those moments, a whole new world opens up. Be mindful of the thoughts that interfere with our ability to spot movement. Be mindful of the voices calling us to attention instead of allowing our eyes to lead the way to relaxation.

Exercise 2.4: Learn to Know a Tree . . . or Two, or Three

Sometimes we don't live next to trees or can't see them out a window. We can go out and explore our neighborhood looking for some trees or any plants, even weeds in a vacant lot. Walking gives us flexibility and has proven power to relieve stress and anxiety. Take advantage of this opportunity to move. Even if we have readily accessible trees, it doesn't hurt to walk to a new location for a change of scenery.

When we get to our destination, we can find a comfortable place to sit or stand. Maybe we'd like to lean against a tree. We need to be still for a few minutes. When we move, we can't see the slower movement of trees very well at all.

Since this is playtime, it's okay to imagine talking and listening to trees. What subjects might interest trees? Wind, weather, insects, birds? Maybe nearby construction that disturbs the ground, this tree's extensive root system, and its connections to other trees' root systems. Does the tree seem happy, excited, calm, or droopy? What might cause those emotions? We don't require scientific proof to play pretend, but for some scientific guidance, read Peter Wohlleben's *The Hidden Life of Trees,* or Robin Wall Kimmerer's *Braiding Sweetgrass: Indigenous Wisdom, Scientific Knowledge and the Teachings of Plants.*

How does it feel to imagine the trees as living, breathing, sentient beings sharing life on this marvelous blue planet? Can we let go of everyday stress in the presence of trees?

Set an Intention and Do It: Practice Daily Forest Bathing

Just as we brush our teeth and clean our bodies, it makes sense to cleanse our mind, spirit, and soul of the stresses and emotions that lead to disease and disability. A daily session with plants and trees can do just this, bringing about both physical and mental health gains.

Exercise 2.5: Set an Intention to Connect with Wood Energy

Changing any habit requires effort from mind and body. We can nurture, motivate, and channel effort by enlisting the spirit of the conscious universe through the compass we created in Exercise 1.2. In this exercise we set our intention by planting a seed instead of writing it down.

1. Get a small container like a clay garden pot, or a paper cup. Make sure it has one or more holes in the bottom for water drainage and fill it with dirt. We can buy a bag of potting soil, reuse the dirt from a potted plant that has died, or dig up a couple handfuls of dirt from outside.

2. Put the container on a plate. Buy a packet of seeds, take something like a bean out of the cupboard, or grab a seed from an outdoor plant. Dandelion seeds work very well! We state our intention to spend time watching the wind blow every day as we plant one seed in the center of the dirt. Push it down the depth of the seed. For example, a dandelion seed would go down about 1/8th of an inch, and a kidney bean would go down about a half-inch.

3. Give the seed some water to dampen the dirt. Put the container in the East on the Compass and visualize this practice growing into a beautiful habit, just like the seed will grow into a plant.

4. Have faith. Check in daily. Give the seed a happy greeting. We're all in this growing game together! Let the seed remind us to practice watching the wind blow. Let the outdoor plants remind us of the life we have planted inside the pot. What can we do to help our sense of playfulness grow and thrive?

5. Keep the faith. If nothing comes up after a week. Put another seed near the first one. Seeds need to meet all their requirements for growth, just as we do. Talk to the seed. What is it missing? Maybe we're missing some of the same requirements as the seed? Perhaps we can adjust our intention to accommodate any insight we receive.

6. Provide the seed with love. Once he or she has sprouted and has a few leaves it will need some sunshine. Put it in a window. Watch the leaves. Our plant will tell us when it needs water and sunshine if we learn to listen with our eyes. In just this way we nurture our intention.

This simple, no-cost practice of watching the wind blow provides the advantages of meditation, immunity boosting, and stress reduction. Find a time of day that works best for spending 15 minutes watching the wind blow. Enjoy doing it with a cup of coffee in the morning or a relaxing beverage after a day of work. Walk to a park or look out a window. Have fun!

Exercise 2.6: Develop a Habit of Daily Forest Bathing

Keep track of daily progress with a calendar that has 1 to 2 inch boxes. Buy something special or use one of the many free calendars that come to us as gifts or promotional materials that we never use. In each box we can write down how many minutes we spent watching the wind blow that day. We can jot down a note about the weather, something we saw, or the progress of our seed. The calendar helps to keep us on track. Worksheet 2.6 provides a blank set of boxes we can use if we don't have access to any other calendars.

Worksheet 2.6: Keeping Track of Progress: Watching the Wind Blow

Write your start date in a corner of one of the boxes in the first row. Continue the numbers sequentially in the boxes that follow until you have filled out 30 days of dates. Each day write down how many minutes you spent watching the wind blow that day. Jot down a note about something you saw, or the progress of your seed.

Sunday	Monday	Tuesday	Wednesday	Thursday	Friday	Saturday

Once we get into a routine, it becomes easier and easier to apply this approach in multiple settings. Feeling stuck in traffic or a checkout line? Watch the trees or shrubs outside move, and let that frustration go. Stymied at work? Take a break at a window, go for a short walk outside, or gaze at a plant on the desk. Even in an office, plants can sometimes catch a breeze. Let stresses go and open up to new possibilities.

Betrayed by a friend? Spurned by a lover? Backstabbed at work? Shocked by bad news? Go outside and shout into the wind. Throw some sticks. Grab a dozen eggs and toss them at trees or rocks. Although we could get accused of littering, the animals and birds will happily accept this offering of extra protein and fat. Birds especially enjoy eating eggs. Let it go. Let it go. Let it go.

Make It Your Own: Practice Weather Watching

Back before satellites and radar, before radio and newspapers, people had a lot more time to watch the sky, the winds, the trees, and the animals. Almost everyone could tell from observation when weather might change for the worse and how to prepare for it. Some people did more watching than others and reached conclusions about what they saw in the world around them, as well as what they felt in their own bodies as weather changed. We know some of that knowledge, and some has been lost, replaced by new knowledge and technology.

Some five thousand years ago, people on the Salisbury Plain of England erected concentric circles of massive stones that align with sunrise and sunset at the solstices. A circle of ancient pits around Stonehenge can accurately predict eclipses. Today we have similar eclipse-prediction abilities and yet still have not completely deciphered how ancients used Stonehenge and the surrounding Aubrey holes, nor how they got the smaller 2-ton bluestones from their place of origin about 150 miles away.

Most of us moderns no longer have time for this level of observation and study, but by spending 15 minutes a day watching the wind blow, we can learn a lot about the world around us. Observe birds, insects, animals, and plants respond to the change of weather and seasons. Jot down what we see in a calendar or journal.

Naturalists have done this for centuries. Charles Darwin developed his theory of evolution, and Gregor Mendel laid the foundations for understanding genetics through keeping just such journals in the 19th century. What insights might we discover with this kind of daily practice?

Can we learn to recognize different species or even different individuals?

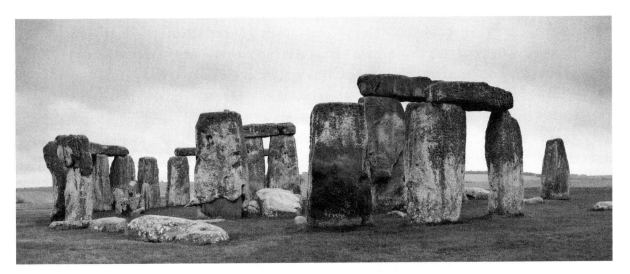

Figure 2.6 Archaeologists believe that Stonehenge was built about five thousand years ago during the late Neolithic period of the "Stone Age." The smaller two ton bluestones were transported from about 150 miles away. Archaeologists continue to argue about whether the stones got there by human or glacial transport.

Doing so sharpens our skills of observation, focus, and attention. Can we learn to predict the weather by observing the behavior of all the species who share our home? Succeeding in these predictions will give us a burst of dopamine.

Like a kid with a deck of cards and a few tricks, we may find ourselves amazing friends and family with our newfound knowledge. Hearing "How'd you do that?" will produce a burst of serotonin.

Dopamine, serotonin, endorphins, and improved immune function—forest bathing can lead us to a whole new level of health and happiness.

Share It: Take a Friend Forest Bathing

Take this practice up another notch with oxytocin. Bring a friend or family member on your next forest bathing expedition. Show them how to watch the wind blow. Relax. Breathe in the oxygenated air, full of immunity-boosting phytoncides, and feel stress, frustration, and anger drift away with the wind. Have fun!

Exercise 2.7: Playing with Children

We live in a culture where children have increasingly restricted access to play, especially outdoor play, and we often encourage children to cut off awareness of their surroundings with all manner of technology from smartphones to computers. Within our culture we have begun teaching mindfulness practice to children. In my opinion, we have other, better options.

Most cultural traditions do not teach meditation practices to children before puberty. These societies allow children plenty of time for play, which relieves stress and encourages awareness and learning. Outdoor play gives children a chance to experience their bodies interacting with our conscious universe. Imaginary play expands life's possibilities and draws on creative resources. Games teach children the three most important aspects of social interaction: how to make rules, break rules, and go along to get along. These types of play form a foundation for meditation practice.

We can take our children to a playground, park, or other natural setting. Sit on a bench or on the grass, and watch children move with the same mindful attention we give to the leaves on a tree. Breathe. Let children explore. Watch what they do. Don't judge. What thoughts and emotions come up? Practice simply observing children's process unless they seem in imminent danger of harm. They will check on us. Nod. Smile. Let them feel our awareness, our mindfulness. Keep breathing. Feel the power of this eyes-wide-open mindfulness practice. Do it often, until it becomes a habit. Including children in our practice of forest bathing can happen on any walk outside. Children notice details that adults have learned to ignore, a bird's feather, an interesting bug, other people's trash. Share children's observations of the world for a few minutes. Ask them about their finds. They can help us connect with wonder.

Deem the minutes we spend following our children as they explore a world full of wonder as eyes-wide-open meditation of the highest order.

Exercise 2.8: Playing with Elders

Most of us keep busy as much time as possible. We do, and do, and do. Take time to be with elders. Sit next to them. Breathe. Speak only when they engage with us. Pay attention to the sounds, smells, and energy of their presence. What thoughts and emotions come up? Breathe. Be with elders. They have unspoken wisdom to share.

Often elders don't get outdoors due to movement limitations or cognitive impairments. Take time to bring an elder outside where he or she can feel the breeze on skin, smell the fresh air, watch birds, clouds, and leaves. For those who have grown up in rural areas, we may find such a trip triggers an elder's lost or long-buried memories. Take time to listen to these stories about another time and place. Elders have wisdom and knowledge we need.

Simple games like checkers, Scrabble, and cards require little expense and often provide a big reward of happy hormones. Sometimes, elders with fairly significant dementia can remember the rules to these games once they feel the cards or playing pieces in their hands. I often play Solitaire with elders. We work together to figure out where cards go and it improves not only cognitive function, but finger dexterity and social skills as well. Using simple games like these can give children a way to relate to and help a grandparent.

CHAPTER 3

Water Energies

Imagine! The Healing Power of Sleep and Dreams

A ruffled mind makes a restless pillow.

—Charlotte Brontë

COLD AS ICE. Hot as steam. Everywhere. Gentle as a mist or cleansing as a tidal surge. Nourishing rain and purgative tsunamis. Eternal mystery. Home of mermaids, leviathans, Godzilla, and Atlantis.

We know less about the deep sea than outer space, yet we trace our origins to both. Shape-shifting water floats as a solid. Steamy water coats leaves with dew, blankets the landscape in fog, rises to the clouds, and returns to earth as mist, rain, snow, sleet, and hail. Water has the power to burst pipes, carve grand canyons, and transform parched brown desert into all the colors of a rainbow.

SLEEP
Bone, Joints, Teeth
Kidney – Bladder
Hearing & Ears
Pain, Temperature, Rocking
SPACE – SOUL
Fear & Moaning
Winter, Evening, Cold
Black, *La-A*
Salty
WATER

Figure 3.1 Life Aspects Associated with Water Energies

Liquid water penetrates everything, sliding through the smallest of openings, dissolving all manner of metals to create the salty oceans that give our planet both life and its blue color. Steam, rain, and ice purify water and give it back to us in as life-sustaining sweet streams, rivers, and lakes. Great masses of ice at the north and south magnetic poles hold water in reserve like massive, antediluvian banks.

Water makes up 60% to 70% of our body, lubricating our joints, regulating our body temperature, and flushing out wastes. Water dances to the waxing and waning of the moon, and those of us who dance with her and howl at the moon like wolves, we call lunatics.

Exercise 3.1: Make a Conscious Connection to Water Energy

Fill a glass with water. Add some ice. What do you notice about water when it floats? Put a pan of water over heat and watch the steam rise. What do you notice about water when it rises? Watch raindrops and snowflakes fall from the (Metal) sky. What happens when there is too much water? What happens when there isn't enough? What do you know about water? Search for some water stories, like accounts of floods in many myths and legends. What can your observations teach you about water? Does water speak to you? Can you talk to water?

Practice: Imagine! A Peaceful Night of Sleep

Just as our lives depend on water, they also depend on getting enough sleep. Virtually all sleep studies agree that we need to sleep a minimum of 7 to 8 hours in each rotation of the earth. Sleep restores the body and soothes the mind. Dreams connect us to a conscious universe in ways we can't always understand, but scientists, inventors, and artists of all mediums confess that their greatest works often began with a dream.

In his book, *Why We Sleep: Unlocking the Power of Sleep and Dreams*, sleep researcher Matthew Walker attributes the following health benefits to sleep:

- A long and happy life
- Better memory and less risk of dementia
- Enhanced creativity
- A slim, attractive appearance
- Relief from food cravings
- Fewer colds, and
- Less risk of heart attack, stroke, cancer, or diabetes.

Our practice for this element on the Healing Compass revolves around preparing ourselves for that life-sustaining 8 hours of sleep every night. To do so we will separate ourselves from our ever-so-distracting electronic media devices. Their blue light and constantly flickering screens keep us alert and awake through our visual system.

Screen refresh, the time it takes an electron beam to scan over an entire screen, happens at rates of 60 to 600 times per second. When that rate drops below 72 Hz we may notice a flicker, but beyond that we may not be aware of any movement, although those energetic frequencies may stimulate the brain in ways that we don't yet know (Morisson, 2015; Cytowick, 2015). Giving ourselves several hours of "down" time from electronics before getting into bed makes sleep much more likely to happen.

How Sleep Heals the Body

Sleep researchers tell us that our sleep has many stages and phases. They organize these types of sleep into two main groups, REM, or rapid-eye-movement, dream states and NREM, or non-rapid-eye-movement, deep sleep states. NREM sleep has four different levels, and each has different effects on the brain and body. All types of sleep positively impact health. They generally occur in 90-minute cycles throughout the night. We have longer sequences of the deeper NREM cycles in the earlier part of the night, between 11 p.m. and 3 a.m., and longer lighter NREM cycles and dream-filled REM cycles between 3 a.m. and 7 a.m. (Walker, 2017) (Figure 3.2).

According to Walker, NREM sleep shows up in MRI measuring equipment as slow waves that ripple across the cortex from the front to the back. Thousands of neurons all fire at the same time to create these waves. REM waves look almost identical to the random spikes and valleys of the awake brain, except that in REM sleep we have no voluntary muscle tone; the body goes limp. The thalamus, in our limbic system (see Chapter 2 – Figure 2.3) cuts off sensory processing during NREM sleep so that we lose consciousness. In REM sleep the thalamus reengages sensory processing, but replays memories, motivations, and emotions in the parts of the brain that would process those sensations. Sleep research tells us that when we are awake we receive sensory information. NREM sleep moves that information into memory, and REM sleep integrates those memories.

In his book, Matthew Walker cites all of the earlier mentioned benefits of sleep. He believes that sleep can truly give us a long and happy life. As a sleep researcher and professor of neuroscience and psychology at University of California, Berkeley, he can back up these beliefs with scientific research.

We know that as obesity rates have soared over the past three decades, our health has declined. Sleep directly impacts our cravings for sweet and starchy foods. A number of books on nutrition, such as Robert Lustig's *Fat Chance* and Mark Hyman's *Eat Fat, Get Thin,* mention the correlations between sleep, weight gain, and diabetes. Walker describes a series of studies done by Eve Van Cauter, director of the Sleep, Metabolism and Health Center at the University of Chicago. Her research subjects who only got 4 to 5 hours of sleep at night ate 300 more calories at the buffet table than subjects who got 7 to 8 hours of sleep a night. The first group also raided the free snack machine for an extra 300 calories every night. All those extra calories add up to a weight gain of 10 to 15 pounds a year. Research subjects who lost weight through diet and exercise programs lost more muscle mass than fat when they slept 5-1/2 hours a night. Those who slept 8 hours lost most of their weight in fat (Walker, 2017).

Sleeping only 4 hours a night made research subjects 40% less effective at regulating their blood glucose, and they demonstrated increased insulin resistance with anything less than 6 hours a night (Walker, 2017). Weight gain, poorly regulated blood glucose, and insulin resistance describe the common factors

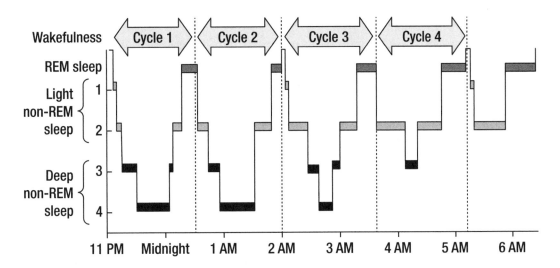

Figure 3.2 Sleep Cycles of 90 minutes occur throughout the night.

that lead to type 2 diabetes and metabolic disease, both of which increase our susceptibility to heart disease, dementia, and cancer (Hyman, 2016; Lustig, 2013).

When it comes to fighting off illness, whether it's flu or cancer, lack of sleep makes getting sick more likely. Walker cites a series of studies on this phenomenon done by Michael Irwin, director of the Cousins Center for Psychoneuroimmunology at the University of California in Los Angeles. Irwin's team found that as little as only one late night and early morning wake-up that resulted in 4 hours of sleep reduced 70% of the natural killer cells that fight cancer for a group of healthy young men.

In 2002 a group of healthy young adults were separated into two groups. Each group received a flu vaccine. In the 6 days preceding the flu vaccine, one group got 4 hours of sleep a night and the other got 7-1/2 to 8-1/2 hours a night. The sleep-restricted group produced less than half the immune response that those who got sufficient sleep did. Even more telling, those people on the restricted sleep schedule did not bounce back to their previous immune levels even 1 year later (Walker, 2017).

Getting enough sleep also improves our odds with cancer. Several large studies on 25,000 to 75,000 people showed increased risk of cancer for those who slept less than 6 hours a night compared to those who got 7 or more hours a night. In part this may relate back to increased sympathetic activity (as in various responses to a threat from Chapter 2). Sleepless nights trigger stress and inflammation. Cancer cells seem to thrive on inflammatory responses to stress as these attract increased blood flow to tumors (Walker, 2017). Shift work, especially irregular hours, appears to have associations with increased cancer risk strong enough for Denmark to pay compensation to nurses and airline personnel who contract breast cancer (Wise, 2009).

Our bodies signal us to slow down and sleep when we get tired right before catching a cold. Instead of drinking more caffeine, taking medications, and "toughing it out," we might have fewer sick days by spending one or two extra days in bed, before we start showing symptoms like a runny nose or sore throat. Aric Prather and his research team found that cutting back on sleep even one night reduced their subjects' resilience to a flu virus sprayed up their nose (Prather, Janicki-Deverts, Hall, & Cohen, 2015). In another study, after six nights of 4 hours of sleep, other subjects showed half the expected reaction to vaccines for flu and hepatitis B (Prather et al., 2012).

The adrenal glands on the kidneys produce three stress hormones, adrenaline (also known as epinephrine), cortisol, and norepinephrine (also known as noradrenaline). The brain also makes norepinephrine, which it uses to transmit information. Hormones get secreted by glands and send information via the bloodstream, whereas neurotransmitters communicate from neuron to neuron. Biochemically many hormones and neurotransmitters are almost identical. These three biochemicals get called into play whenever we face a situation that may require fight-or-flight responses. It can take hours to return the body to its previous state, and during this time heart rate and blood pressure get elevated, putting stress on blood vessels, especially those that supply the heart. When we spend time ruminating on that situation, our bodies can call up those hormones all over again. It's this kind of chronic stress that causes inflammation and tissue damage the body attempts to repair with cholesterol. Plaque builds up in arteries, causing atherosclerosis that leads to heart attacks and strokes (McBride, 2008).

Just one night with an hour's difference in sleep makes a noticeable change in risk for heart attacks and strokes. In fact, every spring, when we turn our clocks forward and lose an hour of sleep, incidence of heart attacks increases the following Tuesday. In the fall, when we turn the clocks back and get an extra hour of sleep, incidence of heart attacks decreases the following Monday (Kanterman, Juda, Merrow, & Roennenburg, 2007).

Drowsy driving may be the most dangerous of all sleep-deprivation outcomes, causing over a million car and truck crashes each year, more than crashes caused by alcohol and drugs combined. We often believe we can make up sleep or do just fine with a few days of less than optimal sleep time. Like the intoxicated driver, sleep-deprived drivers grossly underestimate their impairment, and problems with concentration can begin after only 15 hours of being awake.

Driving after a few short nights of sleep appears to cause the same effects as back-to-back all-nighters in terms of the number of microsleeps that occur. Microsleeps last only a few seconds, long enough to cross from one lane to another at 30 mph. Intoxicated drivers have slow reaction times; people driving during a microsleep have no reaction at all.

David Dinges directs the Unit for Experimental Psychology at the University of Pennsylvania, where he is chief of the Division of Sleep and Chronobiology. He and his fellow researchers there have spent time looking at what happens to concentration after less-than-optimal sleep. They have found that going 10 consecutive days with only 6 hours of sleep, or 6 days of 4 hours of sleep a night, both produced the same number of microsleeps as going without sleep for 24 hours. Their research subjects who slept 4 hours a night for 10 consecutive days had microsleep episodes similar to subjects who had not slept in 48 hours. They also found that three full 8-hour nights of recovery sleep were not sufficient to make up for six short nights (Walker, 2017).

Sleep also plays a large part in successful evolution, inasmuch as looking good to potential mates enables us to pass our genes on to another generation. Tina Sundelin at the University of Stockholm had research subjects rate people's basic attractiveness, in terms of health, tiredness, and looks. Half the women in question were photographed after 8 hours of sleep and the other half after 5 hours of sleep. Both groups were photographed at the same time of day, with the same lighting conditions, and wearing no makeup. Not surprisingly, those who got their "beauty sleep" got higher ratings for attractiveness and desirability as a social partner (Sundelin, Lekander, Sorjonen, & Axelsson, 2017).

Beyond the ability to attract potential friends and mates, reproductive function also suffers from lack of sleep. In *Why We Sleep*, Matthew Walker summarizes studies that show women who get suboptimal sleep suffer from menstrual problems, lowered fertility, and miscarriages in the first trimester of pregnancy. Men who don't get enough sleep fare even worse. A week of sleeping only 5 hours a night will lower men's testosterone levels, giving them an age profile 15 years beyond their actual age. Over time, sperm counts also go lower and testicles get smaller (Walker, 2017).

Going deeper, Walker reports that researchers find lack of sleep ages chromosomes and disrupts those genes that regulate cholesterol, specifically those that regulate HDLs.

This may be sufficient information to ensure committing to 7 or 8 hours of sleep a night. But wait . . . there's more.

Dreams, Memory, Mood, and Creativity

Sleep also affects our mind and quality of life. The slow, synchronized brain waves of deep NREM sleep appear to help us move our memories from short-term storage in the hippocampus of our limbic system to the parts of our neocortex specific to memory for information as well as sensation and movement (see Figure 2.3 to see these structures). In fact, in multiple studies, research subjects who got an opportunity to sleep in between learning new facts and skills did much better than those who did not when it came to later testing. Even short, 20-minute naps made a difference. When researchers further investigated, they found that this type of memory consolidation seemed linked to the kind of Level 2 NREM sleep that lasts longer in the morning hours from 3 a.m. to 7 a.m. (Walker, 2017).

Considerable research indicates that all-night study sessions significantly decrease our ability to remember information on a test. In fact, getting a good night's sleep or even taking a nap before testing will likely improve our scores on any memory-retrieval test. Athletes, musicians, and other people who develop skilled-movement memories through repetitive practice also benefit from sleep. Practicing a difficult set of movements and following that session with a nap or a good night of sleep will improve skill performance (Walker, 2017).

Our dream-filled REM sleep plays an even more interesting part in memory. REM sleep shuts down our production of norepinephrine so that we can replay traumatic memories without their accompanying emotional baggage in our dreams. Dreams seem to have the ability to cleanse us of depression and anxiety that often persists after a trauma. A sleep research pioneer, Rosalind Cartwright spent most of her career examining dreams and dreaming. During her many years at Rush University she explored how REM sleep changes after trauma or with anxiety and depression.

Based on Cartwright's research, Matthew Walker began exploring how specific types of REM sleep help us overcome trauma. Cartwright had found that people had no identifiable depression a year after a traumatic event when they dreamed about those specific, painful events soon after they happened. Walker believes that these content-specific nightmares enable people to revisit traumatic events in an attempt to cleanse their memories of emotion. Often, continued high levels of stress hormones block some individuals' ability to achieve healthy REM sleep. Murray Raskind, from the U.S. Department of Veterans Affairs, who was treating patients for high blood pressure, found that reducing his patients' norepinephrine levels also resulted in the resolution of recurring nightmares for veterans with PTSD. These two men have collaborated in their research findings and continue to explore treating PTSD by encouraging healthy REM sleep (Walker, 2017).

We generally have more REM sleep in the hours between 3 a.m. and 7 a.m., so getting those dream-rich hours of sleep takes on more importance, especially when going through difficult times in our lives. Reducing stress levels for several hours before going to sleep will contribute to healthy REM sleep. Our practice for this chapter specifically targets reducing stress before bedtime.

Dreams enhance our creative abilities. Many creative geniuses have woken from a dream with some of the most important discoveries in modern times. In 1869 Dmitri Mendeleev, a Russian chemist who had spent years trying to find some order to the known elements, fell asleep after a long session of struggling to find some logical uniting thread. In his dreams the swirling elements snapped together into a grid we now know as the periodic table of elements. He awoke and drew the entire table of 63 known elements, only needing to make one correction later. His table's ability to predict the characteristics of newly discovered elements still works today (Popova, n.d.) (see Figure 5.2).

A number of famous people have also dreamed up works that we know very well. Musician and former Beatle Paul McCartney wrote "Yesterday" directly after waking up (Vincent, 2015). Another rocker from that era, Keith Richards of the Rolling Stones, wrote "Satisfaction" while dreaming. Richards recorded an eight-note riff and the words "I can't get no satisfaction" before dropping his pick and falling back to sleep. He filled the remainder of the tape with snoring (Hutchinson, 2013).

In 1818 Mary Shelley birthed the entire genre of science fiction when she wrote *Frankenstein* following a dream tale she'd shared with friends in 1816 (McGasko, 2014). Seventy years later another nightmare caused Robert Louis Stevenson to write *The Strange Case of Dr. Jekyll and Mr. Hyde.* (Ezard, 2000).

Thomas Edison claimed to only sleep 4 hours a night, but he napped in his lab to take advantage of what he called "the genius gap." He slept in a chair with armrests, holding onto several ball bearings. As he began dreaming, his hand would go limp and drop the balls. The resulting sound woke him up so that he could immediately record his dream ideas on an easily accessible notepad (Walker, 2017).

REM sleep produces some amazing creative abilities. Matthew Walker and his colleague Robert Stickgold devised a series of experiments to showcase this. They awakened people from REM sleep and asked them to perform anagram puzzles, also known as word scrambles, and found their subjects solved these better than they did when awake. They also performed much better than subjects awakened from NREM sleep (Walker, 2017).

Walker also discusses a number of other research experiments done to test how REM sleep helps us consolidate and integrate learned material so that we can use that integrated memory to solve complex mathematic and grammatical problems at a later date. Ullrich Wagner at the University of Lübeck in Germany had participants labor over hundreds of number-string problems, performing something like long division for over an hour. If that wasn't frustrating enough, Wagner made it more so by giving participants a set of rules for solving the problems and withholding information about a hidden rule that made solving all the problems much easier. Twelve hours later, all the subjects had to return for another round of problem solving. At the end of the second session the researchers revealed the hidden rule. Only 20% of the group who stayed awake and had time to think about the problems found the hidden rule, whereas 60% of those who had a full night's sleep, including the precious morning REM hours, found the hidden rule on their own (Walker, 2017). The moral of Wagner's study: It really does help to "sleep on it" when solving complex problems.

Another study mentioned by Matthew Walker focused on the disruptive effects of alcohol on REM sleep and consequently learning. Although many of us choose to have an evening drink to relax us and make us sleepy, it turns out to have just the opposite effect. Alcohol definitely sedates us, but after imbibing, we generally have our sleep disrupted by frequent awakenings throughout the night. Alcohol especially suppresses REM sleep.

In the study, Walker describes a large group of students who were divided into three groups. All the students had to learn an artificial grammar similar to computer coding on the first day, and they all learned it with about 90% accuracy. A week later the students returned for testing to see how well they remembered what they had learned. One group had no alcohol during the week and they not only remembered what they had learned, but actually did better after a week of good sleep. The other two groups got a little drunk on a two- to three-shot vodka-and-orange-juice cocktail, precisely calibrated to their weight and gender. The group of students who had their cocktails on the first night after they learned the artificial grammar forgot 50% of what they learned. The group of students who had their cocktails on the third night after learning forgot 40% of what they had learned (Walker, 2017). The moral of this study: Don't drink during your college years—and good luck with that!

Exercise 3.2: Tapping Into the Creative Reservoir

Think about how the universe speaks to us most powerfully. Do we enjoy drawing, writing, singing, playing music, dancing, knitting, or engaging in some other creative endeavor? Set aside some time (15 to 30 minutes) to enjoy doing that. Try doing it in the morning on awakening or in the evening while relaxing before going to bed. How does it feel? Which feels best doing it in the morning or in the evening? Does it get into our dream life?

Sleep Changes Through Life

Our sleep patterns change as we move through life. Before birth we apparently spend almost all of our time asleep. By the end of the second trimester we spend 6 hours of time in something that resembles NREM and the same amount of time in REM sleep. During the other 12 hours, our fetal brains appear to be in some sorts of mixed-sleep types that also do not resemble true wakefulness. By the third trimester we seem to wake up for a few hours a day. Our REM sleep ramps up to 9 hours a day, and by the final week before our birth we hit our lifetime maximum of 12 hours a day in REM sleep (Walker, 2017).

Spiritual healers often speak of the importance of dreams and attribute the time we spend in utero as a time when the universe "downloads" all the information we will need to complete "our contract" during this go-round in Earth school. Sleep scientists describe this as a period of critical brain maturation, a time when neural pathways and connections grow at incredible rates. These pathways connect the cortex, limbic system, and brain stem, enabling the complex associations like those Stephen Porges describes in his polyvagal theory.

Sleep has been an important part of our evolution for about 600 million years. In multiple animal studies, including those of long distant ancestors such as worms, fruit flies, Zebra fish, and rats, active sleep, similar to REM sleep in human newborns, allows geneticists to examine the evolutionary importance of sleep. All of the above animals spend lots more time in active sleep during their early lives. When researchers deprive them of this sleep, all sorts of problems with social relationships and other functional behaviors develop (Kayser & Biron, 2016).

Along these same lines, Majid Mirmiran and a team of researchers found that when newborn rat pups were prevented from active sleep by administration of drugs that are known to interfere with REM sleep, the rat pups had noticeable changes in brain development as adults, particularly in the neocortex (Mirmiran et al., 1983). Daniel Siegel attributes reflection, relationship, and resilience to our neocortex. Researchers also found that even after these newborn rat pups were allowed to make up REM sleep, they never quite managed to make up the difference in their brain development (Walker, 2017).

One might imagine that human infants deprived of REM sleep in the womb and after birth might exhibit problems affecting their ability to react to environmental stress as well as initiate and maintain social relationships. Research on people with autism spectrum disorders (ASD) shows problems with mood regulation, social interaction, and disturbed sleep. They also do not have the marked day and night rhythms indicated by melatonin levels, and they have 30% to 50% less REM sleep when compared to typically developing children (Cohen, Conduit, Lockley, Rajaratnam, & Cornish, 2014).

Children and adults with ADHD also exhibit many of the problems associated with lack of sleep: inability to maintain focus and attention, learning disabilities, behavioral problems, and moodiness. Many of these people have sleep disturbances that often get magnified by stimulant medications, which increase attention but make sleeping even more difficult. Caffeine, the most common stimulant present in beverages, candy, and snack foods, also disrupts sleep, primarily NREM sleep. Many children and adults consume caffeine in processed beverages and foods.

Sleep plays a big role in brain maturation. Infants and children need much more sleep than adults. Newborn infants continue to have large amounts of REM sleep compared to older infants and children. A 6-month-old infant divides the typical 14 hours of total sleep equally between dreaming and deep sleep. Infants and young children typically sleep for many short periods throughout the night and day as they establish their circadian rhythm. The circadian rhythm for adults shows up as a rolling wave line in Figure 3.3. At 1 year of age children's brains have matured and they can sleep for longer stretches at night with one or two naps during the day (Walker, 2017).

By 4 to 5 years of age children can usually sleep 9 to 10 hours a night with just one daytime nap to meet their average of 11 hours. Children at this age generally spend about 70% of that time in deep sleep. Older teenagers and adults divide their sleep into about 80% deep sleep and 20% dreaming (Walker, 2017).

In infancy we need to establish lots of connections between all parts of our nervous systems, and dream-filled REM sleep seems to make that happen. As we get older we need to organize what we learn and get rid of those connections that we no longer need. Deep NREM sleep seems to make that happen. As adults we continue to organize and streamline our neural connections. Throughout life, increases in deep NREM sleep precede our developmental milestones, whether these are crawling, walking, or learning to exercise good judgment as an older teen and young adult.

Our sleep patterns modify as we grow into adulthood. For a brief period of adolescence our circadian rhythm actually changes. Teens tend to feel sleepy later in the evening than most adults, whose bodies generally let them know that it's time for bed at 10 or 11 at night. Teens typically don't feel that urge until much closer to midnight. This also means they tend to get their very important Level 2 NREM memory sleep, and mood-soothing REM dreams, between the hours of 5 to 9 a.m. and wake up grouchy and confused before then. School and work schedules interfere with these important sleep times and often serve as a constant source of friction between teenagers and adults (Walker, 2017).

As we reach adulthood our circadian rhythm shifts back to the typical, familiar adult pattern in Figure 3.3. In 1938 two early sleep researchers, Nathaniel Kleitman and Bruce Richardson, established this internally generated biological rhythm by spending 32 days in the complete darkness of Mammoth Cave in Kentucky (Kleitman, 1952).

Support and Release: The Healing Power of Water Energies

Dreams reconnect us to that mysterious, watery world before birth. Creativity resides in this space of infinite possibilities that some people also refer to as "soul." We come to this life full of possibility, and over time we let some of these opportunities flow away, while we concentrate on what matters most to us at the moment. Our health, our memory, and even our DNA depend on reconnecting to this dream world during sleep.

Beliefs create thoughts.
Thoughts create emotions.
Emotions create actions.
Actions create health.

If we *believe* that sleep is optional, we might *think* of it as something to ration like a forbidden food, *fearing* that we don't have enough hours in the day to accomplish everything we need to do. Cutting sleep hours too short could make us increasingly moody and forgetful, and cause us to lose our vitality and creative drive. Eventually we might find ourselves prone to colds or on the way to various other inflammatory conditions.

When we *believe* sleep is a welcome restorative, we *think* about how to make time for it to do its magic. By getting enough sleep every night we may *feel* our moods improve, feel our creative energy find expression, and even feel less troubled by colds and allergies.

The aboriginal peoples of Australia honor a complex concept that has been translated by Westerners as Dreamtime. The original words from aboriginal languages translate into English as a variety of concepts. These include such ideas as "originating from eternity," "everywhen," "uncreated," and "nonordinary reality." Like many other societies, aboriginal peoples share dreams in public forums through art, music, and dance (Hume, 2004). Sometimes communities respond to these "dreams" by adopting sweeping changes based on those dreams. Indeed, though we often deny a "soul connection" through dreams, Mendeleev's Periodic Table, and Edison's light bulb have created great changes in our modern culture, as have many other dream-originated discoveries, inventions, art, and music.

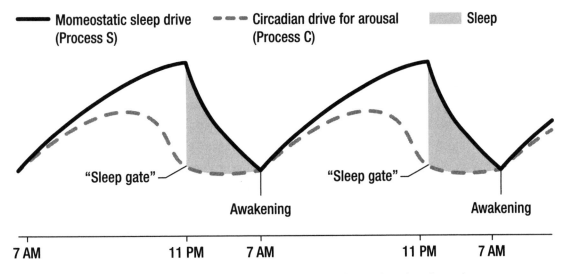

Figure 3.3 Normal circadian rhythm and sleep to wake cycles showing when we are most likely to feel a pressure to sleep or a drive for arousal

Edison's light bulb directly impacted sleep by illuminating the night, something that has led us to later sleep times and health-damaging night shift work. Fear, the emotion associated with water in the Healing Compass, plays a big role in our reluctance to let go of waking consciousness for the frankly delusional and hallucinatory world of dreams. Indeed, keeping a night-light on during sleep probably dates back to humans falling asleep to the dying embers of a campfire. According to many archaeologists our control of fire originated about a million years ago (Gowlett, 2016), so it should come as no surprise that our toddlers often insist on having a little light on at bedtime.

The Healing Compass associates hearing with water, as well as bones, teeth, and joints. We often think of water in terms of sounds: waves, ripples, drops, and crashes. Our ears are the only sensory organ that has bones in it. When sound waves hit the thin membrane of our eardrums its sends those vibrations along to activate three tiny bones shaped like a hammer (*malleus*), anvil (*incus*), and stirrup (*stapes*). These bones send vibrations along to a snail shell–shaped tube (*cochlea*) where fluid transmits vibrations to the cochlear nerve. The nerve's 30,000 fibers pick up that information and carry it to the brain stem. The brain stem sorts out any emergencies that need immediate attention and moves information on to the limbic system, which connects it with memories, emotions, and body needs so it can send that specific set of information on to the parts of the cortex that know what to do with it. One of these networking connections brings us the soothing qualities of music. A steady "heartbeat" rhythm and melodic tones both set off a host of responses that calm us and make us more ready for sleep.

Water resonates with the kidneys and bladder, which purify and store water. Unless bacteria has traveled all the way to the kidneys from the outside world (a very difficult journey), our urine is sterile. Our bladders can stretch. Holding our urine as long as possible from time to time helps to exercise the bladder and keep it elastic. This also strengthens the muscles of our pelvic floor to make it possible to hold on longer. Therapists recommend *kegel* exercises to help clients develop the kinds of strength and flexibility we need to make it through an entire night of uninterrupted sleep.

Many of our joints contain fluid, and all of our bones and joints have lots of nerve endings that warn us about damage through pain. When we listen right away, we minimize that damage. When we "push through," we sometimes cause more damage. Often, especially as we get older, we fear that a pain indicates a lifelong affliction. Joints and pain generally respond well to warmth, although many health practitioners recommend cold for initial, traumatic injuries because it slows down inflammation. Treating our aches and pains by loving them up with some TLC in the form of a bath, hot pack, or capsicum (red pepper) creams will go a long way toward relieving pain and allowing the joints to heal. A warm bath will help us sleep and take advantage of sleep's power to heal.

We sleep better in the dark, but live in a constantly illuminated world. Black-out curtains, eye pads, and turning down the lights 2 hours before bedtime will help both children and adults get ready for sleep. People used to sleep longer hours during the dark winter nights before the 24-hour clock became so influential in factory work.

The slow, wave-like motions of a rocking chair, a swing, or dancing put our

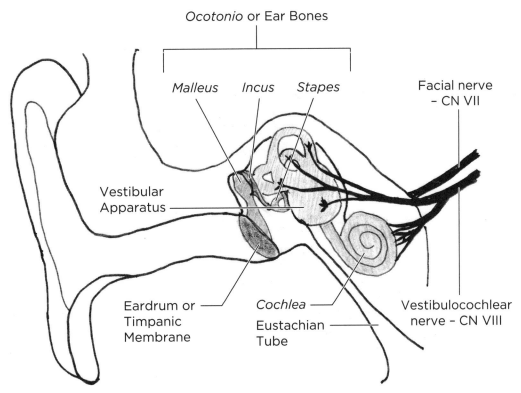

Figure 3.4 Anatomy of ear showing the three ear bones (*ocotonia*) and cochlear nerve. Mechanical sound waves move the eardrum which passes the movment through to the *Malleus*, *Incus*, and *Stapes* activating nerve endings in the *Cochlea* that send these energetic messages to various parts of the brain for interpretation and response.

bodies into a more relaxed state. These activities associate with Water energy and call us to Sleep.

Imagine! Dream Your Way to Health

Who has time for sleep? With so much to do we don't seem to have enough hours in the day. Like play, sleep often falls off the end of our very long "to do" lists.

Worrying triggers our "monkey mind" to ruminate over not falling asleep, the ever-so-long "to do" list, and a myriad of other issues, which activates Earth energies (see Chapter 4). Earth energy can stop or slow down the flow of Water energy that carries us into sleep. Our crazy schedules mean we eat late at night, and digestion activates more Earth energy that slows our journey into dreamland.

Nightly calls to the bathroom (insufficient Water energy) wake us up and interrupt our sleep time. Restricting fluids for a few hours before bed can help

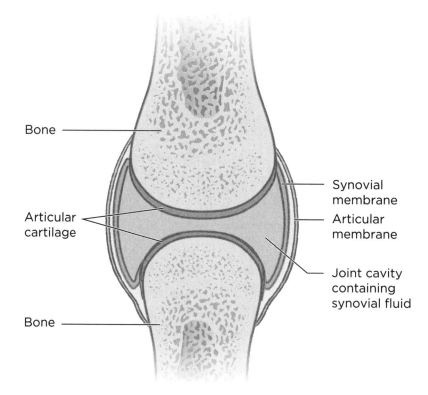

Bone

Synovial membrane

Articular cartilage

Articular membrane

Joint cavity containing synovial fluid

Bone

Figure 3.5 The majority of joints in the body contain fluid for smooth movement. Joints have nerve endings which primarily convey sensations of pain and temperature to the brain.

with that. Salt, the flavor of Water energy, affects water retention in the body. In hot climates, people often increase their salt intake to maintain hydration because salt holds onto water in our bodies. Salt can affect our blood pressure by increasing the total volume of water in our bodies.

Salt cravings may represent our bodies' need for more water, or more Water energy. Getting enough sleep also meets those needs and can affect our cravings for salt. Getting up frequently during the night to urinate can reflect salt intake during the day. Pay attention to how salt intake during the day affects the need to empty our bladder at night.

Stress (insufficient or erratic Wood energy) can play a role in night sweats that wake us up. Taking time to play, to relax, and nurture ourselves helps to strengthen Wood energy.

Our practice for Water energy focuses on improving sleep by turning off all electronics for 2 hours before bedtime. Even watching television can put our bodies on alert because of its flickering images and bright light.

If we use electronics to play solitaire, check our social media accounts, or answer emails to manage anxiety and relax during the day, the alerting effect of the screens works to our advantage. In fact, using blue light during the day can actually help keep us awake and help us feel more fatigued at night when we need to sleep (Viola, James, Schlangen, & Dijk, 2008).

Blue lights at night have a counterproductive effect. The incredibly bright blue light of computer screens (even when dimmed) alerts the nervous system and tells us to wake up. Blue light has an alerting effect dating back some 500 million years to when we emerged from the seas that blocked everything but blue light (Rosbash, 2003).

Putting a blue-blocking screen on our devices or wearing yellow glasses after sunset might alleviate some of the problems of alerting blue light, but it does nothing to stop the automatic screen refresh that generally happens so quickly we don't even notice it. Our eyes can process movement much more rapidly than we used to think. We can thank the computer gamers for this information, as computer games and monitors strive to go beyond human capabilities in order to provide realistic images. Our visual system alerts us to movement because that, more than anything else, indicates a predator approaching. Thus, the movement of the scanning electron that generates a screen refresh may not register as a flicker, but it may stimulate an alerting fight-or-flight response in our nervous system.

Beyond the mechanics of view screens, what we often watch on television and social media involves stories that can trigger fight-or-flight responses. Think about the amount of violence we see in shows or on the news. Marketing specialists often tell advertisers to sell products by finding and triggering the "pain" or "fear" point. Are your teeth white enough? Is grandma going to fall down and not get up? Is gluten making you sick? Do you need to take a medication? Tell your doctor . . .

Pharmaceutical ads not only suggest that we need a medication for a condition we may never have known existed but also spell out in rapid detail all the possible dire outcomes that taking this medication will cause, generally including death.

All of these types of information trigger stress responses that block sleep. Turning off electronics 2 hours before bedtime will help reduce the amount of stress we take in before we want to go to sleep.

Our auditory system will alert us to unusual sounds, and sleep researchers have found sleep cycles disrupted by sounds that did not result in full wakefulness. Sleep specialists recommend a sleeping area free of media, with low lighting, blackout curtains, and white noise to drown out the odd sounds that might disturb sleep, especially in areas of high traffic (National Sleep Foundation, n.d.).

Exercise 3.3: Try Disconnecting from Our Media

We need to provide ourselves with an 8-hour opportunity to get essential amounts of sleep each night. That means we need to do some math.

1. How much time do we need in order to get done what we need to do (eat, groom, dress, and care for others) before heading out the door in the morning?
2. What time do we need to wake up to make that happen?
3. Subtract 8 hours from that time to decide when it's time to get in bed.
4. Then subtract another 2 hours to decide when it's time to turn off the electronics.
5. Begin turning off electronics a full 10 hours before you want to wake up.

What to do instead? Imagine our ancestors laughing at this question.

- We can read.
- We can listen to music or audio books.
- Try drawing a picture, coloring, knitting, or making something you've put off because you haven't had the time.
- Try doing yoga, tai chi, qigong, meditation, or another slow moving, relaxing practice you enjoy.
- Take a bath. Harness the power of Water to calm the body. The temperature change of getting out of a warm bath helps make us feel sleepy (Walker, 2017).
- Play cards or board games. Try solitaire with real cards again!

Exercise 3.4: Learn What Makes Falling Asleep Easier

Sleep research has contributed a lot of information about how to support good sleeping habits. Here's a list of the top recommendations from sleep researchers about what they call "sleep hygiene." See what techniques work best for you.

1. Make a schedule so that we can go to bed and wake up at approximately the same time each day. Keeping to a schedule strengthens our circadian rhythm, our internal clock that tells us when to sleep and when to wake up.
2. Avoid taking stimulants such as tobacco, caffeine, and alcohol close to bedtime. As our bodies metabolize these drugs that often causes us to wake up in the middle of the night.
3. Progressively dim the lights as it gets closer to bedtime. Sleeping in darkness seems to help a lot of people. Try an eye mask or room-darkening shades to see if that helps with getting a good night's rest.
4. Make the bedroom a quiet space. Use earplugs or white noise to help out when we can't change our larger environment.
5. Make the bedroom a sacred space, a space set apart for sleeping, cuddling, and making love. Keep it clean and uncluttered. (Read more about decluttering in Chapter 5: Metal Energies.) Choose a mattress, pillows, sheets, and blankets that feel comfortable. Add a plant or two

to purify and oxygenate the air. Keep electronics out of the bedroom as much as possible.

6. Engage in calming activities in the hours before bedtime.

Reading in bed often proves a great way to ease us into sleep. Reading scary stories or the news can trigger stress responses, but although we read using our eyes, our brains process those words in the more calming auditory processing parts of our brains (Porges, 2011). That means we can sometimes fall asleep while reading murder mysteries, thrillers, and newspapers. As any college student knows, textbooks can put us to sleep almost instantly.

Reading print on paper will put us to sleep faster than looking at a backlit screen. As of this writing, nothing definitive has surfaced in the research about "paper white" screens or LED lights on the side or in front of a screen. If we struggle with insomnia or falling asleep, it might be safer to stick to print-on-paper formats.

Taking a warm bath before bed also helps relax our bodies. The warmth of the water raises our core temperature. When we get out of the bath into the cooler air, our bodies begin to cool down, especially our hands, feet, and face. Sleeping in a cool room, from 55 to 65 degrees Fahrenheit (13 to 18 degrees Celsius) helps us relax into sleep. Warming our hands and feet with gloves, socks, or a heating pad, surprisingly enough, acts to lower core temperature and lulls us into sleep (Walker, 2017).

Set an Intention and Do It: Practice Getting to Bed on Time

Sleep restores body, mind, and spirit. Like life-giving water it keeps us alive. Under ideal conditions, we can live only about three days without water to drink. We can survive somewhere between 10 days to a month without sleep. Prolonged sleep deprivation causes brain damage and massive organ failure. (Walker, 2017). Sleep must include dreaming to connect us to the creative reservoir of the conscious universe. We need dreams to help us process emotions. Getting to bed and providing ourselves with an adequate amount of deep sleep and dreaming may be one of the most important things we can do to stay healthy.

Exercise 3.5: Set an Intention to Connect with Water Energy

Changing any habit requires effort from mind and body. We can nurture, motivate, and channel our efforts by enlisting the spirit of the conscious universe through the compass we created in Exercise 1.2.

1. Pour water into a special glass or cup and place it in the North position of our Healing Compass.

2. Contemplate the water. Where did it come from? Think about all the places it travelled to get to us. All the water on our planet stays here, to nourish us and give us life. Who else has drunk or bathed in our water? Imagine some of the molecules of water coming to us carrying the energy of those we love, our ancestors, the men and women of history and legend who went before us. Imagine dinosaurs and all the plants and animals who came before us drinking and bathing in our water. Water connects us to life itself.

3. Remember a time in our life when we felt ALIVE! Full of creative energy and connected to all of the life around us. Perhaps we were with a lover, a parent, or a child . . . Perhaps we were immersed in a creative project or deep in the woods, the ocean, the desert? See that time. Feel it. Hear it. Smell it. Taste it. Connect it with an intention to get enough sleep every night.

4. We can hold this memory as an intention while we drink our glass of water.

5. Let that memory seal our commitment to give our minds, bodies, and spirits the time they need to replenish, rejuvenate, and restore our health and resilience. We can repeat this exercise whenever we want, or even every night.

6. Doing this between the hours of 3 pm and 7 pm takes advantage of Water energy's strongest time during the daily cycle AND means we're less likely to have that glass of water wake us up in the middle of the night!

Exercise 3.6: Practice Getting to Bed On Time for a Month

Make a schedule that provides a full 8-hour opportunity for sleep every night. We calculated which hours work best for us during "Try it Out," and now we commit to following that schedule for a month so we can really assess how getting enough sleep affects us.

Hopefully, we have worked out some of the kinks that come along with such a rescheduling of our lives. Here's a list of the ones that most of us encounter. Spend a few moments thinking about to deal with these sleep challenges as they arise.

- *Get all work that requires a backlit screen done at least 2 hours before bedtime.* In Chapter 5 we'll discuss why we bring work home and how to change our beliefs, thoughts, and emotions about what Work means to us. For now, clear a 2-hour window for relaxation instead of work before bedtime.

- *How will we interact with friends and family members who might object to our earlier bedtime?* If we're used to watching a screen or spending time on social media with others, how might we manage that time differently? Can we turn off our phones for the night? What else might we do to stake out this time and space for our health and still enjoy our friends and family?

- *What pursuits will provide relaxation for those 2 hours before heading to the bedroom?* Some of us relax when we know we have everything ready for the next day. Making a "to do" list or packing our lunch provides peace of mind. Take time for self-care with massage. Engage in some of the creative activities from Exercise 3.2. Enjoy a warm bath. Connecting with the conscious universe through prayer, meditation, or contemplating nature can also ease us into the world of dreams

Keep track of the time spent in bed (our sleep opportunity), what we did to prepare for sleep, and the quality of sleep we had with a journal, a calendar or Worksheet 3.6.

Worksheet 3.6: Keep Track of Progress Getting to Sleep On Time

Write your start date in a corner of one of the boxes in the first row. Continue the numbers sequentially in the boxes that follow until you have filled out 30 days of dates. Each day write down how many hours you spent sleeping before waking up that day. Jot down a note about what you did to prepare for sleep on the previous night. Give your quality of sleep a number grade from 0-5. 0 equals no sleep. 5=delicious sleep & dreams. Use the back of the sheet to jot down dreams you remember.

Sunday	Monday	Tuesday	Wednesday	Thursday	Friday	Saturday

Make It Our Own: Practice a Bedtime Ritual

We take what we have learned from this month of practice to create a personalized bedtime ritual. When do we have that last soothing cup of warm tea? Which lights do we turn off first? Which lights stay on? How much darkness brings the best sleep? Do we need to get some blackout curtains, or will a simple sleep mask work? Do we sleep better with earplugs or a white noise machine like a fan or something fancier that plays the sounds of rain or waves?

What activities will we choose to occupy our time? Do we vary them or follow a more structured schedule? Is a bath relaxing or more work? What reading material calms us down? Do we have special music, prayer, meditation, or other activities that feel right?

Make the bedroom a sanctuary. Get rid of electronics like a TV or computer when we can, to remove temptation. Keep bed linens clean. Splurge on some special sheets, a blanket, or pillow to make us feel pampered.

Make whatever works best part of a nightly ritual that clearly signals our bodies to prepare for sleep.

Share It: Set an Example

Sleep, like eating and relieving ourselves, falls entirely within our own powers of self-regulation. We cannot control another's bodily processes, even those of our children, in these three essential bodily functions. Nor can others control us. We can simply create a supportive environment, one that provides what bodies need to achieve good sleep, good nutrition, and relaxed elimination. We must take care of ourselves and set an example for others. They may join us or not. Often when we focus on our own self-care, we give those we love permission to do the same. Getting 7 to 8 hours of sleep a night can often improve our looks, memory, energy levels, and mood. We'll be more likely to stay healthy and miss out on most of the bugs that go around. People will notice. When they ask about what you do, share your sleep journey and rituals. You could save a life.

Exercise 3.7: Sleep for Children

Children need more sleep than adults. Sleeping in the early days, weeks, months and years of life fosters brain maturation. Adults can benefit from naps, but for children under four or five years of age they are essential. Night and day sleeps provide different types of sleep "nourishment" in much the same way NREM and REM sleep provide different neurological benefits.

Infant brains develop rapidly, and they need more sleep to accomplish brain maturation. As children mature they need less sleep, but even into the teens and young adulthood increased sleep hours often precede integrating a new skill.

Indeed, for athletes, musicians, and other performance occupations, napping after practice can lead to demonstrable improvements in skills after that nap. According to a variety of sleep researchers and pediatricians:

Newborns need 15 to 16 hours a day, generally in 4- to 5-hour bursts;
Infants need 12 to 16 hours a day, including two to three naps;
Toddlers need 11 to 14 hours a day, including one to two naps;
Preschoolers need 10 to 14 hours a day, including one nap.
School-age children need 9 to 12 hours a day. They can generally skip naps, but may want one during growth or learning spurts. A nap before 3 p.m. never hurts anyone. After that it may make it harder to sleep at night.
Teens need 7 to 12 hours of sleep, but their sleep rhythm will advance forward by about 2 hours during their teen years, which will often conflict with other schedules.

Just as we learn to follow our body's sense of sleepiness (the line that crests like a wave in Figure 3.3) we need to observe what our children do to indicate sleepiness and make sure they get the time they need to sleep. All children will exhibit behavioral and learning problems when they miss out on sleep. Unfortunately, lack of sleep causes increased arousal which means that children will have a harder time going to sleep and this can become an ever-increasing cycle of fussiness and irritability that produces stress hormones that interfere with sleep.

Even more than adults, children need to have a schedule and rituals that set the stage for sleeping. The sleep habits we develop as children will follow us into our teen years and on into adulthood. Establishing good sleep habits as adults sets an example children can follow. Getting enough sleep as parents helps us have more energy and patience to deal with the challenges of sleep-disrupted children. In addition to turning off electronics for two hours before bedtime, the following suggestions help children and adults honor their own sleepiness and make sleep easier to achieve.

- Follow a schedule based on when children become sleepy, and get them to bed early, before full sleepiness, so they can relax into quiet, protected sleep. Make this time consistent, so children establish a personal sleep rhythm.
- Keep electronics, phones, televisions, and computers out of bedrooms. A small night-light and soft music with a 60 beats per minute (heart rate)

rhythm, or a white-noise machine can support sleep rather than interfere with it as electronics do.

- Put children to bed when they feel sleepy, but before they completely fall asleep so they can learn to relax themselves into sleep. Having an adult sitting close by while reading a book or listening to soft music may reassure a child, but all children must learn how to calm themselves into sleep.
- Rocking, reading, singing lullabies, warm baths, massage, and swaddling before bed all help relax an infant or child and get them set to continue their own self-soothing once in bed.
- Sucking soothes infants, and many infants and young children self-soothe with nursing or a bottle before bedtime, and a thumb or pacifier in bed. Avoid bottles in bed, even water. As liquid pools around teeth it provides a perfect medium for bacteria to grow and can result in dental decay.
- Spending 30 minutes to an hour a day in outdoor play will help a child (or an adult) achieve a circadian rhythm that helps regulate both sleep and appetite. Daily outdoor play in a child's schedule is as important as mealtimes and bedtimes.

Exercise 3.8: Sleep for Elders

Often adults don't realize that our sleep has deteriorated, and we attribute many of the signs of sleep deprivation to old age: memory loss; depression; low energy; and illness. Restoring good sleeping patterns can help ameliorate or even reverse some of these changes. Sleeping pills don't restore missing deep NREM sleep and can make getting up from bed to go to the bathroom, groggy and unbalanced, even more dangerous (Walker, 2017).

Older adults change their sleep patterns in the opposite direction of teens, shifting sleep and wake times back an hour or two. Since our body's production of melatonin drives this rhythm, no amount of wishing and trying to stay up actually works.

Many restaurants have "early bird" specials that cater to the earlier rhythms of elders. Go with the flow of your body. We need to get bed earlier and avoid further fragmenting our sleep by trying to "push through," only to wake up on the couch or in an easy chair. Look at that sharply peaked wave of sleep pressure in Figure 3.3. Taking a late nap, or dozing any time after 3 p.m., will make it harder to fall asleep later on. We need to work with our new normal. Go to bed at 9 or 10 p.m. and get up with the birds (or even before the birds in summer!).

And don't neglect that 30- to 60-minute walk outside or even rocking on the porch. Exposure to daylight, even on a cloudy day, will help with melatonin levels. The added exercise will promote sleep as well.

Older adults often begin having disrupted sleep in midlife. We once thought older people just needed less sleep, but many research studies show that all adults need between 7 and 8 hours of sleep a night. Work schedules, children, increased needs to use the toilet at night, medical conditions, and the pharmaceuticals prescribed to treat those conditions all play a role in disrupting adult sleep. Generally speaking, adults first lose their deep, restorative NREM sleep. Sleep waves get smaller and less powerful and this tends to continue incrementally as we move through the decades. Often we rely on alcohol and sleep medications to increase our sleep time, but both of these old standbys actually anesthetize us instead, decreasing our amount and quality of REM sleep (Walker, 2017).

CHAPTER 4

Earth Energies

Eat What You Love! Don't Worry. Feel Better.

Worrying is using your imagination to create something you don't want.

—ESTHER HICKS

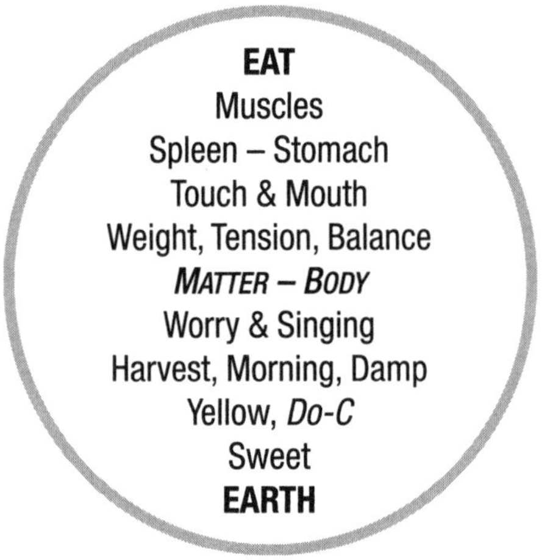

EARTH ENERGY RESONATES with the dirt beneath our feet, decomposing organic and inorganic matter, home to worms, microbes, mushrooms, Hobbits, and trolls. Created from the interaction of water dissolving rock and the appearance of life on this planet, as life morphed into death, organic matter collected, got deeper, richer, and full of abundant life.

Dirt nourishes us. Plants come from the soil and their roots hold the ground in place so that all Earth creatures have somewhere to make a home. Earth gives generously. Earth's season, midsummer, abundantly bright with sunflowers, tomatoes, squash, and corn, includes all the hard work that goes into harvesting them. Everyone I know who has given up or cut back on gardening did so because they could not keep up with harvest's abundance. Earth's energy is strongest in the morning (from 7 a.m. to 11 a.m.), a time for hearty breakfasts and sharing stories over brunch.

Earth has a shadow side, too, earthquakes, mudslides, famine—times when

EAT
Muscles
Spleen – Stomach
Touch & Mouth
Weight, Tension, Balance
MATTER – BODY
Worry & Singing
Harvest, Morning, Damp
Yellow, *Do-C*
Sweet
EARTH

Figure 4.1 Life Aspects Associated with Earth Energies

she strikes suddenly or withholds her bounty, and fortunes change. Abundance of thought, food, and companionship has a flip side of worry, overthinking, over-planning, and obsessing about "what if . . ."

We can soothe these anxieties with Earth energy as well. Singing, using our muscles, massage, and staying in balance all resonate with Earth energy. So does heading to the kitchen for a snack, preferably something sweet, because that flavor resonates with Earth energy, too.

Eating is the daily habit that brings Earth energy into our lives. We receive her bounty through our mouth and stomach. Our spleen and other glands supply enzymes that prepare food for digestion, aided by descendants of the very microbes who evolved from those first life forms, friends we have carried with us in our digestive tracts all our lives. They enable us to transform food (matter) into body, mind, and spirit.

Exercise 4.1: Make a Conscious Connection to Earth Energy

Grab a handful of dirt or mud. Draw your fingers through some dust and grime. What do you have in common with these substances? We are all creatures of this planet and we come from its, dirt, dust, mud or what have you. Search for "Creation Stories" and you will find many that connect the creation of humans with the element of Earth.

Practice: Eat What You Love! And Detox from Sugar, Flour, and Alcohol

We receive a tremendous amount of food, information, and emotions every day. Some of it nourishes us and some of it does not. How do we focus on what helps us to thrive? All sorts of detoxification protocols exist, and more come out every day. Many of these require us to throw out all the foods in our cupboard and replace them with unfamiliar and often expensive substitutions. When these additions to our diet taste bad to us, it's almost impossible to stay the course for any length of time, regardless of the health benefits they promise.

The detoxification practice in this chapter costs nothing extra and might even save some money. We will focus on eating foods that taste good and nourish our body, mind, and spirit, while eliminating the three most common and addicting food-related toxins—sugar, flour, and alcohol.

Day by day, as we loosen their addictive hold over us, we make room for other delicious and nourishing foods to take their place. Usually, cravings for sugar, flour, and alcohol disappear within days, replaced by positive changes in mood, energy, and clarity of thought we hadn't believed possible. This practice increases our awareness of how what we eat affects our health and empowers us to choose those foods that sustain us, for pleasure as well as nutrition.

What Happens When We Eat

After chewing and swallowing food, our stomachs break it down further with acid that destroys dangerous microbes, protecting us from disease. As food leaves our stomach, important enzymes from the spleen, liver, gallbladder, and pancreas get added in to further break down what we have eaten so that we can absorb food's nutrients through our small intestines.

Microorganisms in our stomach and small intestine help us digest some of the foods we eat. In the large intestine, or colon, even more microorganisms complete the process of sorting out and distributing what will nourish us and preparing what won't for elimination. By the time what we eat has made it through the digestive tract, our bodies have transformed whatever entered our mouths into immediate energy, stored energy, valuable body tissue, or waste. Our gastrointestinal system both nourishes us and protects us from harm.

Nutritionists divide foods into three basic macronutrients: fats, proteins, and carbohydrates. We need to eat proteins and fats in order to receive essential fatty acids and amino acids that our bodies cannot make on their own (hence *essential* for life). All people need enough protein and fat to maintain long-term survival. Carbohydrates provide fiber and essential micronutrients, such as vitamins, minerals, and phytonutrients.

Essential micronutrients in carbohydrates, as well as those in proteins and fats, serve important functions in our bodies, but because we need micronutrients in such small amounts it rarely serves us to try and regulate our health through them. Supplements in the form of vitamins, minerals, phytonutrients, and probiotics have become a very lucrative industry. However, most research studies show that simply eating a balanced diet of fats, proteins, and carbohydrates (in the form of fruits, vegetables, and grains) will maintain vigorous health unless you have a very extraordinary metabolic disorder.

A few indigenous groups of people actually have thrived quite well primarily on animal fats and proteins, supplemented by vegetables and fruits, with little or no grain-based foods. The Masai in Africa and Inuit in the Arctic Circle are two examples (Price, 2008). Hearing about these groups has led many people to adopt low- or no-carbohydrate diets. If we have descended from Masai, Inuit, or a similar ancestry, we will probably do well on a no-grain diet. If we come from almost anywhere else on the planet, we generally won't sustain a low- or no-grain diet without a lot of willpower and good motivation (such as regaining our health after a serious diagnosis). This chapter focuses on pleasurable eating and sharing nourishing food with others. To do this we must enjoy the way our food looks, feels, smells, and tastes.

"Eat what you love," does *not* mean eat anything you want. It means tuning in to what we eat, refusing to put into our mouths anything that tastes bad, and exploring a variety of foods to find more foods we like. We also need to *love what we eat* and choose foods that love us back by providing us with nutrients we can use. We want to eat when we feel hungry, as that heightens our senses. Waiting until we feel a sense of starvation or deprivation generally leads to overeating or binging. We evolved by listening to our bodies, and when we relearn this way of eating we regain our balance with food.

Demystifying Calories and Nutrition

A thousand years ago we didn't worry about food choices. We ate what we could get, and that varied by season. In temperate regions like Europe and North America, eating seasonally meant leafy greens, milk, and eggs in spring; fruits, vegetables, cheese, and eggs in summer; root vegetables, nuts, grains, and meat in fall; bone broths, grains, nuts, cheese, and other fermented (preserved) foods in winter. Honey was hard to get and highly valued. Maple sap appeared in early spring, just as food stores dwindled (Kimmerer, 2015), and cane sugar was virtually unknown outside India and the Persian Empire. A lot has changed since then.

When we talk about nutrition we generally refer to the three macronutrients—

fat, protein, and carbohydrates—that provide almost all of the nutrients we need to survive. Fats and proteins provide building blocks for all the tissues and organs that make up our bodies. Carbohydrates provide fiber and micronutrients. Fiber helps protect the lining of our intestines and moves food more effectively through them. Micronutrients, small amounts of vitamins, minerals, and colorful phytonutrients, contribute to our overall health.

We also count calories. Dietary information has relied on the long-standing and well-defended myth that "a calorie is a calorie." Inasmuch as the term "calorie" refers to a standardized scientific measurement for the amount of heat it takes to raise 1 gram of water 1 degree Celsius, this statement holds true.

Since the middle of the 19th century, nutrition researchers have measured the amounts of heat that each food produces when burned under controlled conditions in a laboratory. Doing so provided a basic and standard measurement of potential energy contained in food products (Nestle & Nesheim, 2012).

It will probably come as no surprise to hear that what happens to food in a controlled laboratory and what happens in our digestive tracts bear little or no resemblance to each other. The three macronutrients become useful sources of energy through different digestive pathways, and this makes a lot of difference in their usefulness to our bodies.

Over millions of years, our digestive systems have developed elegant ways of keeping us supplied with energy and the means to create body tissues. These systems have multiple feedback loops that will keep us going through feast or famine. We can eat a whole lot of junk, or next to nothing, and still not only survive but also often thrive.

Imagine throwing a load of grass clippings into the car and trying to drive. It won't even start. Our bodies won't survive long on grass clippings either, but bodies store energy in all kinds of places, including fat cells, and we could manage to get around the block quite a few times before coming to a halt having eaten nothing but indigestible grass.

In order to understand how we get energy from food, let's imagine a balanced meal of the three basic macronutrients, protein, fat, and carbohydrates, where each portion equals 100 calories. To make the meal more fun, let's add a cocktail, 1-1/2 ounces of 80-proof vodka in 8 ounces of orange juice. On our plate we have 3 cubic inches of steak, 3 cups of steamed broccoli topped with a cubic inch of butter, and 1/2 cup of plain white rice. Each ingredient equals 100 calories. In Table 4.1 we can see where all of those calories go in our bodies.

Table 4.1: Where Have All the Calories Gone

100 Cal Serving	Glucose	Fructose	Protein	Fat	Digestion	Brain	Liver	Raises blood glucose	Raises blood triglycerides	Insulin required
1½ oz. 80-Proof vodka					10	10	80	Yes	Yes	No
8 oz. Orange juice	53	40	7		10		50	Yes	Yes	Yes
3 cups Broccoli	65	7	24	4	10		10	Yes	Minimal	Yes
½ cup White rice	91		9	1	10		16	Yes	Minimal	Yes
3 cu. in. Steak			82	18	25		15	Minimal	Yes	Minimal
1 cu. in. Butter			1	99	3		96	No	Yes	No

Let's start with the cocktail. Vodka contains ethanol, which is the fun part of wine, beer, and spirits. Ethanol has no macronutrients. Vodka, like other distilled spirits, contains primarily ethanol, so it has no nutrients.

Beer, wine, and other fermented beverages contain ethanol as well as carbohydrates from the grain, fruits, and even in some cases milk that served as the basis for their fermentation process.

As we can see from the Table 4.1, in the Digestion column, digesting our drink takes about the same amount of effort (i.e., calories) to digest as most foods. Our brains get that special little thrill that comes only from ethanol. The remaining 80 calories, devoid of any nutritional value, go straight to the liver, where they take one of two potential energetic paths:

1. Immediate energy used by small intracellular structures called mito-chondria, which transform matter (i.e., nutrients) into the energy that powers every cell in our body. Almost all cells have some mitochondria, but cells that have to do a lot more work have more than others. Our livers work hard and have 1,000 to 2,000 mitochondria in each cell. Even with those large numbers, when we eat and drink too much we can over-whelm our liver's ability to manage. We can see in the chart that alcohol, orange juice, and butter send the largest number of calorie-producing nutrients to our livers. The liver uses some of those calories to do the work of making . . .

2. Stored energy, generally sent as triglycerides to fat cells in our liver and muscles. Too much fat in our liver or muscle cells makes it harder to process glucose in our blood, creating insulin resistance, and over decades, fatty liver disease and cirrhosis.

The fun calories of ethanol that go to our brain stimulate our happy hor-mones, dopamine, serotonin, and endorphin, which make us want more, and more, and more.

Our meal has three carbohydrates, juice, broccoli, and rice. Carbohydrates consist of sugars, starches, and fiber. Like ethanol, carbohydrates need an average amount of calories to get digested. Only a small portion of calorie-producing nutrients from broccoli and rice go to the liver for further metabo-lism, but orange juice sends a whole lot more because it naturally contains sugar.

Starches, like the rice, consist of glucose molecules connected together in chains of varying sizes. Sugars consist of three types of single molecules—glucose, fructose, and galactose—that combine together to create double mol-ecules of sugar. Fructose tastes sweet like fruit. Glucose tastes sweet like plain rice. Galactose tastes sweet like fresh milk.

Sucrose, which occurs naturally in ripe fruit, can be extracted from plants like sugar cane and beets. It tastes sweet because it contains one molecule of fruc-tose and one molecule of glucose. Appendix A, "Sugar by Many Other Names," describes many of these molecular combinations of sugar and gives their com-mon names. Fructose gives fruit that tasty sweet flavor. Ripe fruits have many micronutrients, and fructose cues us to eat lots of them during their generally short growing seasons. Like ethanol, fructose stimulates happy hormones, mak-ing us want more, and more, and more.

Many carbohydrates, like the broccoli, also contain fiber, which provides no calories. Fiber comes in two types, soluble like the pectin we add to juice when making jams and jellies, and insoluble like the peelings of fruit and vegetables or the strings in celery. Both of them help us digest our food, and they only occur together in whole fruits, vegetables, and grains. This gelatinous fiber matrix fills the stomach and turns off our hunger hormone (ghrelin) so we stop eating (Lustig, 2013).

Supplements generally give us soluble fiber, which does little good without stringy insoluble fiber to hold the soluble fiber in place. The matrix of soluble and insoluble fiber we get from vegetables, fruits, and grains coats the lining of our small intestines, which slows the absorption of nutrients. It also speeds up movement of what we ate through our digestive system, so food gets to the colon faster. That triggers another hormone (PYY) that tells us we have eaten enough (Lustig, 2013).

We can't digest fiber, but the industrious microbes in our colon love it. These microbes help us further digest food, break down toxins, and take good care of our immune system. We need lots of fiber to keep those microbes going, especially when they have to compete with sugar-loving microbes for real estate in our intestines.

Of all the carbohydrates in our imaginary meal, only broccoli has any fiber. Orange juice, like all juices, contains no fiber. Blending and juicing vegetables and fruits breaks down their fiber into small enough particles that they no longer get digested as fiber. Thus, juice and smoothie carbohydrates consist solely of sugars, starches, and micronutrients. White rice, and any grain that has had its brown outer covering polished off, contains much less fiber than it would ordinarily have. Grinding grains into flour also diminishes their fiber content to varying degrees (Lustig, 2013).

Every cell in our body can use glucose once it gets into the bloodstream. Rising levels of glucose in the blood stimulate our pancreas to release insulin. Insulin plays many roles, including letting our brains know that we have had enough to eat. It does this through several pathways that decrease both hunger and pleasure. Insulin also promotes storage of glucose as glycogen, a harmless starch that keeps glucose out of the bloodstream and makes it readily available when needed for metabolism.

Excess glucose gets converted to triglycerides that generally move to subcutaneous fat cells living under our skin, rather than to fat cells around major organs like the liver and heart, where fat can do more harm than good.

Orange juice sends more calories to the liver because all of the fructose calories have to go there to get metabolized. Too much fructose:

1. Overwhelms liver mitochondria because fructose takes three times more energy to metabolize than glucose.
2. Increases insulin resistance, which means cells can't absorb the glucose they need for energy. This causes the pancreas to make more insulin, and that causes more triglycerides to get stored as fat cells around the liver and other organs, which can contribute to heart disease.
3. Sets off various inflammatory processes that contribute to accelerated aging and "leaky gut" syndrome (damage to the intestinal barrier that allows bacteria and abnormally large molecules to enter the bloodstream). It also produces uric acid, which can stimulate increased blood pressure and gout (Lustig, 2013).

Like ethanol, too much fructose depletes the liver and causes the pancreas to work overtime because of increased insulin resistance. Fructose also blocks signals to the brain from hormones (leptin) that let us know we've had enough to eat. Fructose bypasses our sense of "I feel full and happy." Instead, after eating sugar, we still feel hungry (starving!), and need to eat more for both pleasure and satisfaction (Lustig, 2013).

Extra insulin in our blood appears to drive the growth of cancer cells. Increased insulin resistance correlates with increased risk for dementia, and has caused a number of physicians and nutritionists to refer to Alzheimer's disease as type 3 diabetes (Lustig, 2013).

Fiber mitigates the harmful effects of fructose because it slows down our metabolism. Eating whole fruits, with all their fiber intact, slows down digestion so that the liver has more time to metabolize the nutrients it receives, sending triglycerides and glucose to the bloodstream at a steadier pace.

Our 3 cups of broccoli have plenty of glucose, very little fructose, and about 10 grams of fiber. Three cups (three cups!) of broccoli will just about fill our plate. The broccoli's 10 grams of fiber fulfill about one third of our recommended daily intake of 30 grams (U.S. Department of Health and Human Services, U.S. Department of Agriculture, 2015). Imagine eating three full plates of broccoli every day. This may seem like a lot, but estimates from scientists who study what our hunter-gatherer ancestors ate tell us that they possibly consumed 10 times more fiber than we do today! (Hamley, 2014).

White rice consists mostly of starchy glucose. It takes insulin to help our bodies store the glucose it doesn't use right away. The liver needs to do very little work to metabolize white rice. If we eat so much we can't store it as glycogen, then the excess gets converted into triglycerides in the liver. Insulin levels can spike with 1/2 cup of white rice, but unless we have diabetes, all that broccoli fiber will probably work its beneficial magic, slowing down absorption to a manageable amount. That means less excess glucose in the bloodstream, and less insulin released to store extra glucose as fat.

Diabetes, Insulin Resistance, and Obesity

Diabetes affects more than one in 10 Americans, according to a 2017 report from the Centers for Disease Control (CDC). They predict these numbers will rise. Only 5% of these people have type 1 diabetes caused by genetics and auto-immune destruction of beta cells in the pancreas. The other 95% have preventable or lifestyle-dependent type 2, "insulin resistant" diabetes.

Type 1 diabetes usually affects children and young adults when the beta cells stop producing enough insulin to process the glucose in their blood. On the other hand, type 2 diabetes has a direct correlation with the ratio of body fat to muscle, so it often accompanies obesity. One out of four Americans over the age of 65 has type 2 diabetes. We used to think of this as a disease that affected only elders, however, as childhood obesity rates have risen, so has pediatric type 2 diabetes. According to the CDC, diabetes affects about 2 in 1000 children under the age of 18. This number has risen steadily over the past decades and will probably increase as childhood obesity rates increase. Diabetes and obesity most frequently affect those with less money and fewer social opportunities. Both these factors correspondingly limit food choices and opportunities for recreational activity.

Our bodies have very elegant and complex ways of ensuring that we have enough glucose and insulin. The pancreas produces insulin all the time and stores it for quick access. Excess glucose in the blood causes inflammation. With diabetics, long-term inflammation from excess blood sugars results in debilitating circulatory problems such as loss of sensation in the feet and hands (neuropathy), blindness, amputations, heart attacks, and kidney failure. Diabetics can't release stored insulin, because they don't have enough beta cells to make it (type 1) or keep releasing it as fast as they make it because cells can't use it (type 2) (Bernstein, 2011).

Although scientists have conflicting opinions about how cells become resistant to insulin, most agree that cells become more sensitive to insulin again when we stop eating high calorie, high carbohydrate diets and increase our physical activity. We need a medical practitioner to diagnose insulin resistance and diabetes, but we can change the way we eat and move to prevent or reverse insulin resistance today.

What About Fats & Proteins?

Proteins have 22 amino acids our bodies use to make 50,000 other proteins into neurons, muscle, skin, organs, and virtually every other tissue in our bodies. We need to eat 9 of these amino acids, because we cannot produce them in our body. Animal proteins (meat, fish, poultry, dairy, eggs), as well as quinoa, buckwheat, hemp, chia seeds, and spirulina algae, contain the full complement of these 9 essential amino acids, so we call them complete proteins. Mixing rice and beans, beans and seeds, and nuts and grains will provide all the essential amino acids, even when not eaten at the same meal.

As we can see from Table 4.1, steak takes a lot more work (calories) to digest than any of the other foods on our plate, although the liver doesn't have a big job to do. Only the broccoli takes less liver energy to metabolize it. These principles hold true for other proteins and fiber-rich vegetables.

Proteins do not spike blood glucose levels, so they do not overstimulate insulin release except in large quantities (as in "my stomach feels so full!"). Animal proteins (apart from milk) have no carbohydrates, so they tend to keep blood glucose low, whereas plant-based proteins do include carbohydrates and can spike blood glucose, although they also often come with protective fiber that slows down glucose absorption (Bernstein, 2011).

Fats spend the longest time in our stomachs, but their complicated-sounding digestive process takes the least amount of energy to metabolize. None of fat metabolism requires insulin, so eating fats does not affect blood sugar or insulin release (Bernstein, 2011).

Fats melt in our mouths (the yum factor) and easily slide into our stomachs. They keep us alive by providing us with essential omega-3 and omega-6 fatty acids. Our mitochondria can use these fatty acids as well as glucose to produce energy. We use fat's triglycerides and cholesterol to make cell walls, hormones, neurons, and the protective myelin sheaths that wrap around neurons, empowering them to transmit information more rapidly and effectively. Our bodies store excess triglycerides as subcutaneous or visceral fat in times of plenty.

We generally find more omega-3 fatty acids in animal foods (fish, seafood, and grass-fed meats and poultry) and omega-6 fats in plant foods (vegetable oils, nuts, and grain-fed meats and poultry). Fats don't dissolve in water and cannot enter the bloodstream until they become water soluble. Our stomach, liver, and gallbladder all work together to transform fats into fatty acids. Fatty acids and monoglycerides combine to form triglycerides that join with cholesterol and other molecules. All these compounds travel through the lymphatic system to the bloodstream.

Differences in the molecular bonds of saturated, monosaturated, polyunsaturated, and trans fats create different end results in the blood stream. Although nutritionists continue to argue over the benefits of saturated and unsaturated fats (both butter and steak have saturated fats), they all agree on problems with trans fats also known as partially hydrogenated fats.

Early in the 20th century, chemists found that they could keep fats from going rancid by partially hydrogenating them. They did this first to make a substitute for lard in laundry soaps. Later these same manufacturers marketed their stable fat for baking, frying, and margarine (Forrestal, 2009). When fats go rancid they release free radicals that damage cells. Trans fats don't go rancid for years and years, which makes them popular for processed foods that spend a long time on grocery shelves. Foods like butter, cream, meats, and vegetable oils have a short shelf life, measured in days and months rather than years. Unfortunately, the extra-strong bonds that connect trans fat molecules cause other problems. Trans fats have been linked to abdominal weight gain, heart disease, and insulin resistance (Hyman, 2016).

Neurons, hormones, and myelin enable our brains and bodies to function. Stored fat cells make the difference between life and death in times of famine. Seasonal periods of famine occur even in the best of times. All around the world, cultures celebrate rituals of both feasting and fasting. Our bodies have multiple feedback loops that enable us to conserve fat, and understanding this goes a long way toward explaining why it's so hard to lose weight on any diet. In spite of fat's currently bad reputation, eating fat and having subcutaneous body fat contribute to overall health (Tara, 2017).

What Makes Us Get Fat?

Eating to lose weight seems like an oxymoron. Yet all diets prescribe such a regimen. Not eating, or not getting enough nutrients from what we eat causes us to lose weight. Although weight loss has become the holy grail of modern life, for most of our time on this planet adults maintained stable weights throughout their lives. Only famines or disease caused weight loss and up until just a few decades ago, plumpness indicated health.

Our bodies know how to manage occasional feasting, but frequent overeating overwhelms our mitochondria. Extra ketones in the blood (from metabolizing fatty acids) get disposed of in urine, which can deplete the kidneys over time. During lean times, glucose in our blood drops, with a corresponding decrease in insulin, and lower insulin triggers the body to break down stored triglycerides for energy. Anytime we reduce blood glucose our bodies automatically begin to metabolize fat, starting first with the fat stored around organs. Too much glucose and too much insulin means we don't burn fat.

Most of us have tried lots of diets and exercise regimens that promised we would lose weight. Most of us have failed, not because we don't follow the regimen, but because our bodies do everything they can to hold on to fat cells. Physiologists have begun referring to fat as a highly evolved and protective organ system. We need it to stay healthy and protect ourselves during times of famine (Tara, 2017).

The "gold standard" diet of weight loss, eating fewer calories than we burn off in exercise, has proved particularly misleading and heartbreaking, because we don't burn that many calories in exercise. Most of the daily calories of energy we use come from simply breathing in and out, digesting our food, maintaining our temperature, and otherwise getting through the day. The fraction we burn exercising makes very little difference compared to our overall metabolism while just sitting still (Nestle & Nesheim, 2012).

When we follow a diet that reduces calories below our daily needs, we trigger our famine responses and go into starvation mode. Biochemically, starvation makes us feel lazy and grouchy. Add in strenuous exercise and our body goes all out to hold onto every fat cell it can. Once our metabolism shifts into famine/starvation mode it rarely shifts back, so now it takes fewer calories to maintain weight. This physiologic truth is the reason why almost every diet fails to produce long-term weight loss for almost everyone who tries them. As soon as we begin eating as we did before we regain our previous weight, and usually a little more (Hyman, 2006).

The good news is that physical activity helps. Movement increases the number of mitochondria we have to burn energy. Physical activity also increases endorphins, those happy hormones that give us an exercise high. Physical activity decreases stress and depression. Physical activity increases insulin sensitivity, so we need less insulin to process glucose. Movement increases our feeling of satiation, having enough to eat, by stimulating the hormone leptin. Movement helps us lose the more dangerous fat cells that have collected around our organs.

Even 15 minutes a day will do the trick. We can walk, dance, run, lift weights, do housework, mow the lawn, plant a garden, shovel some snow, swim, or play with our dogs and kids. All of this activity builds extra muscle, reduces stress, and makes us feel satisfied. It likely won't change our weight more than a few pounds. We need to get comfortable with our weight, our muffin tops, and our thighs. Eat less. Make more nutritious food choices (cook at home and eat fewer convenience foods). Keep moving. Have faith in our body's ability to take care of us. Keep it simple. Spend more time feeling happy and energetic and less time worrying about a number on the scale.

Eating and Our Minds: Why Are We So Anxious About What We Eat?

In this country, blessed by so much abundance we throw away almost half of all the produce we buy (Gunders, 2017), how can we have food anxiety? Yet we worry endlessly about what to eat. Did we get enough of this or that micronutrient? Is gluten hurting us? What about dairy? It seems like our news and advertising media have a new food scare to tell us about almost every week. Of course we end up anxious about food.

I don't know about you, but when I feel anxious, I often stop by the refrigerator or the shelves of my local convenience store. I'm sure to find some carbohydrate or sweet treat to numb my feelings. Anxiety plays a large role in our food choices, so learning to manage anxiety with movement and other activities provides a healthier alternative to eating, especially eating sweets.

Beliefs create thoughts.
Thoughts create emotions.
Emotions create actions.
Actions create health.

If we *believe* that foods can harm us, we *think* more about what we've heard about a food's properties than how that food tastes or smells. We may avoid eating with friends because we don't know if we can manage to find "safe" foods at restaurants or someone else's home. We anxiously read the fine print on every label or choose to trust the large, and often misleading, branding information. We may *feel* fearful about what's in fresh food, preferring to purchase familiar and safer-seeming processed foods that tell us they are "gluten free," "organic," "fat free," or "sugar free." One thing all nutritionists can agree on is that fresh, unprocessed foods are always a more nutritious choice than anything in a package.

If we *believe* that our amazing digestive systems can handle just about anything in moderate quantities, we *feel* comfortable about what we eat. We learn to trust that our senses of smell and taste will alert us to foods that don't agree with us, sometimes before we take even one bite. Fewer stress hormones such as cortisol and adrenaline interfere with our digestion. We can go out with friends, relaxed in the knowledge that we will surely be able to find foods we can enjoy. When we shop, we buy foods that look fresh and ones that smell and taste good to us. We eat with confidence and competence, and our health reflects our ability to do so (Satter, 2008).

Let's look at the stories behind two of our current food "demons"—fat and gluten. For millions of years people depended on *fat* to keep them alive. Fat is easy to digest, tastes good, and carries a big calorie and nutritional load in a small package. Weston A. Price, a dentist who studied indigenous diets starting in the 1930s, found that all over the world most people got about 80% of their calories from fats. They ate butter in the Swiss Alps, grubs in Africa, whale blubber in the Arctic, and fish and coconuts in Polynesia. He described these populations and how their health changed as processed foods entered their diets. His book, *Nutrition and Physical Degeneration*, first published in 1939, is still in print.

As the incidence of heart disease increased during the 1950s and '60s, researchers began looking at the effects of diet on health outcomes. A British researcher, John Yudkin, looked closely at sugar consumption. Like Price, he concluded it played a role in obesity, dental disease, diabetes, and heart disease. Yudkin wrote a book, *Pure, White, and Deadly,* to bring his findings to the public in 1972. Around the same time an American researcher, Ancel Keys, began studying diet as well. He wrote *The Seven Countries Study,* which concluded that fat, and more specifically saturated animal fats, contributed to heart disease. Both researchers depended on correlations. Keys chose to report on only 7 of 22 potential countries, possibly because the data from the unchosen 15 countries, which included France and West Germany, did not match his hypothesis. The Sugar Research Foundation, funded by the sugar manufacturing industry and major soft drink companies, spent a lot of money to make sure studies like Keys's got lots of media attention, and also paid researchers to critique Yudkin's and similar studies that showed ill effects from eating sweets (Lustig, 2013).

Low-fat dietary recommendations came out on top of that particular food fight. They became encoded in the United States Department of Agriculture (USDA) dietary recommendations, and for the next three decades we embarked on a nationwide experiment, decreasing dietary fat and correspondingly increasing dietary sugar. We have learned that we all got fatter, and many more of us have diabetes. Saddest of all, type 2 diabetes (insulin resistance) that used to plague only adults over 65 has now become a pediatric scourge.

Gluten, the protein in wheat, rye, and barley grains, has also come under fire. Celiac disease affects about 1% of Americans. These people cannot digest gluten, which causes an inflammatory reaction; damage to the lining of the intestines; and absorption of larger than normal, inflammatory molecules into the bloodstream, known as leaky gut syndrome. Although other inflammatory foods such as sugar can also produce leaky gut syndrome, gluten has taken the brunt of dietary criticism. You don't have to have celiac disease to exhibit sensitivity to gluten. In fact, we all have sensitivity to grains, nuts, seeds, and beans.

Plants have spread all over the globe because they have protective enzymes in their seeds that keep them from being digested by animals. In this way animals have deposited plants' seeds on the ground, intact, with fertilizer. If you find eating a slice of whole wheat bread tastes bitter, and it sits like a lump in your stomach, blame it on these plant protective "antinutrients."

Traditional preparations of grains, seeds, and beans have always included several hours of soaking in water before cooking. During this soaking, the grains get "tricked" into sprouting, which neutralizes their antinutrients and makes many more B vitamins accessible for absorption. Whole grain flour benefits from being mixed with wet ingredients and allowed to sit for 6 to 8 hours before baking, because even grain particles get tricked into going through the sprouting process (Pollan, 2013).

When we made the so-called healthy switch from white to whole wheat flour, we forgot that we can't prepare them using the same methods. White flour has its fibrous outer covering and inner germ sifted out. When fiber goes, so do most of the antinutrients as well as some proteins and vitamins. White flour does not require soaking; whole grain flour does. The big problem with flour (of any type) is that it loses much of its beneficial fiber during the grinding process. Whole grain flour retains more of its protective fiber.

Many proponents of the paleo (low-carb or cave-man) diets cite the fact that humans have not had enough evolutionary time to accommodate cultivated grains into our digestive systems. Given that we believe agriculture is only about 10,000 years old and human DNA gets an opportunity to evolve every 20 years or so (during conception) human DNA could not possibly pull off digesting a relatively new food in such a short amount of time. We don't do the hard part of digesting grains, though. We leave that mostly to the microorganisms in our intestines. Microorganisms reproduce very quickly, so their opportunity for adapting to environmental changes happens in minutes, hours, and days. They definitely know what to do with all kinds of foods, and if you feed them regularly with gluten, they'll take care of it for you (unless you have celiac disease). We have to cultivate our intestinal ecosystem with lots of variety to make sure we have all the good microbes we need. Starving them by avoiding gluten (or any other proteins) will surely cause us to have sensitivity to those foods once we eat them again, because the microorganisms that do the job aren't there to help us digest them.

Eating only a few foods exclusively also sets the stage for developing food sensitivities and allergies to those very foods we eat all the time. Our bodies need variety to maintain healthy immune responses to our ever-changing environment. Scientists are only in the beginning stages of recognizing how the microorganisms in our gut communicate with our brains (the gut-brain connection). The more we learn about this two-way conversation, the more complex it becomes. We do know that maintaining a diverse population of microorganisms in our gut has a profound effect on our immune system, and keeps us healthy in many different ways.

In my opinion, the best dietary news of all comes from a research study done in 1977 in Sweden. The researchers wanted to understand why women from Southeast Asia did not have iron deficiencies even though their traditional diet was very low in iron. They gave a group of Thai women and a group of Swedish women an identical Thai meal and found that the Thai women absorbed almost all of the available iron while the Swedish women absorbed much less, because the Thai food was unfamiliar to them. Next they put the typical Thai meal in a blender and made it into Thai mush. They put a typical Swedish meal of ground beef, green beans, and potatoes into a blender and made it into Swedish mush. They gave Thai mush to the Thai women and Swedish mush to the Swedish women and neither group absorbed more than 30% of the available iron, because it looked nasty and tasted yucky. The moral of this study: We absorb more nutrients when the food looks, smells, and tastes good to us (Hallberg, Bjorn-Rasmussen, Rossander, & Suwanik, 1977).

Nourishing the Spirit: Loving Our Food

Nutritional content does matter. We can mindfully and joyfully consume a bag of corn chips or a box of cookies, absorbing every possible nutrient, and still end up with a sum nutritional total of something close to zero, simply because, apart from the calories, these foods don't have much other nutritional value. In fact, their starch and sugar content causes terrific spikes in blood glucose and insulin which, with constant repetition, will do untold inflammatory damage. The result of this damage and the time it takes to develop into noticeable health problems depends on our genetic makeup.

Still, we have to pay attention to that Swedish study. We get more out of our food when we feel good about it. How can we feel better about what we eat and stop worrying about conflicting health benefits, scare stories, and everything else?

1. *Share food.* Sharing food around a campfire has been a human tradition from way before we had agriculture. Children learn what to eat and how to prepare food from watching adults. Many studies show that sharing family meals reduces obesity, improves school grades, and decreases teen pregnancy and drug use (Satter, 2008).

    Family meals mean that everyone shares the same foods, unlike restaurants where everybody gets to order just what they want without having to share. When I work with families who struggle with picky eaters, I recommend that in restaurants parents order one or two entrées, a couple of side dishes, and one or two desserts for the whole family to share. This saves money since most restaurant portions can easily feed a family of four. A large part of our national trend toward obesity has come from supersizing our portions. We can even share food in fast food restaurants, rather than ordering each child a more expensive individual serving that often includes a toy.

2. *Have faith in our body.* We can digest an amazing array of foods because of our gut microbiome. Many diets call for strict adherence to a set of guidelines. This makes it hard to share food with others unless they follow the same diet regimen. Sticking with a program 80% of the time will give us a host of benefits, whereas denying ourselves while watching others eat something we love will likely result in a binge sooner or later (Satter, 2008). As a species we have survived millions of years of feast and famine. Our bodies have amazing resiliency, and the microorganisms we carry with us have even more (Claus, Guillou, & Ellero-Simatos, 2016).

3. *Develop a relationship with food.* Welcome food into our bodies. Cook at home for a broader sensory experience of the food we prepare. Grow something to eat. Herbs and tomatoes require a small pot of earth, water, and a few hours of daily sunshine. Sprouts require only water and attention. Get to know people who provide us with food. Meet farmers if possible and get to know about the lives of plants and animals we eat. Even when we shop in a big box store, we can learn to recognize people who stock the shelves and take our money. Say hello and thank them for their efforts that feed us and our families. Food has essence, a spiritual quality that transcends the material nutrients it provides. Developing a relationship with food heightens its nourishing value (Lu & Schlapowsky, 2015).

4. *Learn to recognize what enough feels like.* We can measure out portions, or we can pay attention while we eat. Look at food. Does it have pleasing colors and shapes? What might make it more appetizing? Does the texture of our food feel good on our fingers and in our mouth? How does it smell? How does it taste? If we don't like it, we don't have to eat it. When do we start to feel satisfied? Usually, even when we have had enough, if the food tastes really good, we want more. Pay attention to that moment. Enjoy a few more bites. Give thanks to the life that we have eaten and the people who brought it to us. Check in again. Did we get enough?

We're used to mindless eating, cleaning our plates and snacking while driving, reading, or watching TV, and staying current with social media. It may take some time to get reacquainted with what "enough" feels like. We need to stop eating when we feel 70% full. When is that? Usually it's the moment in the meal when we ask ourselves, "I wonder if I am 70% full?" I always eat a few more bites after that, and 80% full works just fine, too.

Exercise 4.2: Conduct Your Own Low-Cost Genetic Study

Take a look at some old photo albums. Go back at least before 1970, prior to the development of low cost high fructose corn syrup, an agricultural policy that subsidized farmers to grow plentiful low-cost food (corn and soybeans), and the low-fat recommendations. This trifecta of national policy decisions led to increased sugar in our diets, supersizing our portions, and universal weight gain.

Prior to the latter half of the 20th century we expected adult weights to stabilize after puberty and remain relatively stable throughout our lifetime. Now we expect adults to steadily gain weight, in college, after pregnancies, in middle age. As we leaf through these old photo albums we see body types more in line with our original genetic make-up without the detrimental effects of our contemporary dependence on processed and convenience foods.

Find a relative that looks like you. Check out their body type. Do you weigh more, less, or the same? Height and weight are dependent on genetics. When we see a match for looks, it clues us in to a host of other genetic markers. Ask elders what happened to the health of those who share large parts of our genotype. Pay attention to their health histories, they may predict our own. A great many chronic diseases have definite links to what we eat, and changing our diets for the better can make a difference.

Receiving and Transforming: The Healing Power of Earth Energies

Our muscles have a special relationship with what we eat. When we get too much to eat our body has to store it somewhere as glycogen or fat. Our muscles have thousands of tiny mitochondria in every cell. Scientists believe these mito-chondria were one of the earliest forms of life on the planet. Mitochondria convert glucose and fatty acids into energy for everything that we do.

Exercise, using our muscles, brings some very important health gains. The more we move and stay active, the more muscle we build and the more mito-chondria we have to burn energy. As muscle mass increases, we burn more calories even sitting still (Nestle & Nesheim, 2012).

Different Types of Body Work

Most people have a familiarity with massage as body work, but there are many different styles and types. The list that follows can give you an introduction, although it can't cover every available type.

Acupressure   follows the meridians from Traditional Chinese Medicine, and uses pressure on acupuncture points to release and move energy.

Acupuncture   follows the meridians from Traditional Chinese Medicine and uses needles to release and move energy.

Amma   also follows meridians and acupuncture points, but does so by making small circles rather than using deep pressure. Amma practitioners also use essential oils in their practice.

Chiropractic   by manipulating the spine chiropractors release tension on nerves that "feed" the body, and assist the body in healing.

Cranio-sacral therapy   holds "pulse points" throughout the body to support the healing flow of energy.

Deep tissue massage   seeks to release deep adhesions in muscle tissue for healing. Recipients often find this practice painful as well as helpful.

Lomi lomi   a form of Hawaiian massage uses fists and forearms in wave-like motions.

Myofascial release   uses gentle steady pressure and stretching to release the fibrous connective tissue supporting and surrounding all muscles, tendons, bones, and organs.

Reiki   moves energy around the body for healing through gentle, light-handed or near-touch.

Reflexology   uses thumbs and knuckles to move energy through organ and body parts that have connections to specific correlations on the palm of the hand and the sole of the foot.

Shiatsu massage   recipients remain clothed, and generally lie down on a floor mat to receive treatment from a practitioner who uses stretching and pressure to move energy around the body.

Sports massage   similar to deep tissue massage, this technique focuses more specifically on muscles and joints.

Thai massage   similar to Shiatsu, but may be done on a table or mat.

Therapeutic touch   moves energy with very light-handed or near-touch.

Exercise 4.3: Managing Anxiety without Eating

Anxiety often drives us to eat. Media scare stories about food make us even more anxious about eating. Now we have a vicious cycle of eating and anxiety, eating and anxiety. We can learn other ways to cope with anxiety. The following list provides a few ideas. Try:

- Moving meditations like walking somewhere to watch the wind blow relieves stress and anxiety and helps build muscle mass.
- Massage will relax the tension in our muscles. Get a massage or some other form of body work. Learn self-massage techniques and use them to reduce cravings.
- Singing resonates with earth-energy frequencies. If we're feeling hungry, and think it might be anxiety, we can try singing to relieve cravings.
- Eating a hearty breakfast before 11 a.m. and scheduling smaller meals or snacks at 3- to 5-hour intervals after that helps us eat less.
- Eating early in the day boosts metabolism, and eating on a set schedule decreases food anxiety.

We can try something from this list whenever we feel an urge to eat emotionally, such as when schedules get too busy, deadlines loom, relationships become tense, or the news cycle predicts doom and gloom. Pick something and try it for a few days. Does it help reduce cravings for food? Jot down your experiences in a journal, or on a calendar.

Eat What You Love! And Detox from the Standard American Diet (SAD)

We all have a tendency toward addiction to three foods: sugar, flour, and alcohol. These foods form the mainstays of processed food industries, which include factory farming and all that it entails. These foods also underlie many serious health conditions, such as diabetes, obesity, dementia, and joint inflammation. Our practice avoids the following three foods for long enough to release their addictive hold over our choices.

- Sugar in any of its forms, including honey, agave, and artificial sweeteners (see Appendix B for a list of sugar substitutes)
- Flour in all of its forms, regardless of its origin
- Alcohol in all its forms: beer, wine, and spirits.

By doing this we allow our body to normalize its response to glucose and increase insulin sensitivity. We add more fiber into our diets, and move closer to whole foods, which always have a higher nutrient density than processed foods.

High-fat and fiber foods will help us get over cravings. Nuts make a great alternative. Try some cream (heavy or whipping) in coffee and tea as an alternative to sugar. Instead of simply adding our usual amount of sugar to drinks, cereal, or other foods, try adding one teaspoon at a time and tasting to see if it's sweet enough.

The U.S. Food and Drug Administration recommends eating no more than 10 teaspoons (40 grams) of sugar a day. Most 12-ounce soft drinks have at least 10 teaspoons of sugar added. The same goes for sweet teas from the store. The World Health Organization recommends only 8 teaspoons a day. When we keep track of how much sugar we eat in a day it often surprises us.

A teaspoon contains 4 grams of sugar. When we make our own teas at home we can add just enough sugar to make them taste good. Usually we will find that "sweet spot" long before reaching the amount of sugar that food and beverage manufacturers add.

In *That Sugar Film,* filmmaker Damon Gameau documented a month of eating the FDA's recommended 40 grams (10 teaspoons) of added sugar a day, exclusively from "health" foods. The movie both entertains and shocks as we watch his health deteriorate. Viewing it can definitely make us think a bit more about what eating sugar does to us.

Stop bringing sugar, flour, and alcohol home. We can go ahead and eat the foods already in our cupboards, or give them away. When shopping, read labels on processed foods. If one of the many names for sugar (Appendix A) appears in the first five ingredients on the list, put it back on the shelf. When we don't have these items at home, we don't eat them as often. Sugar, flour, and alcohol become occasional treats, not everyday foods. Occasional sugar, flour, and alcohol won't get us into trouble (unless we already have diabetes). The large amounts we eat daily are what have led us to gain weight and get sick.

Exercise 4.4: Try Paying Attention to Sugar, Flour, and Alcohol

Be aware that when we eat sugar, flour, and alcohol we rarely ever feel like we have eaten enough. Sugar, flour, and alcohol bypass the neurohormonal loop that tells us we've had *enough*. They also trigger hormonal feedback loops that tell us we are hungry; in fact they often make us feel starved! Our starvation feedback loop makes us tired, so we move less. Alcohol and sugar go right to our dopamine-sensitive reward centers in the brain, and that makes us want more. Together, these pathways drive a vicious cycle of cravings, weight gain, and insulin resistance. In contrast, fats and fiber trigger different neurohormonal loops that tell us we've had enough (Lustig, 2013).

Start noticing how often we reach for sweets, flour, and alcohol. What feelings send us in that direction, and what happens emotionally when we begin saying, "No, thank you" if someone offers them?

Use the Basic Nutrition Journal (Worksheet 4.4) to help with this exploration. Each time we have a meal or snack we write down what was eaten and make a quick analysis of how this food breaks down from a nutritional standpoint.

- Portion: How much did we eat? The easiest measuring device is our own hand. It accommodates our body size regardless of age or weight. Any solid food, like steak or pizza, is measured against the size of our palm in circumference and thickness. For instance, a Chicago style thick crust pizza slice and a New York style thin crust pizza slice folded

Worksheet 4.4: Food Journal – Pay Attention to Basic Nutrition

Name:

Start Date: _____   **End Date:** _____

Date	Food Eaten	Portion	Protein (meat, fish, poultry, eggs, dairy, soy, beans)	Fat (butter, nuts, cream, oils, lard, fats from fish, meat, poultry)	Carbohydrate (fruits, vegetables, grains, breads, pasta, cereals)	Nutritional Quality	Emotions and Sensations Noticed Before, During, or After Eating

Nutritional Quality: 0 = alcohol; 1 = sugar; 2 = processed food; 3 = whole food

Portion Measurement /: protein = palm size; carbs = handful size; fats/sugars = distal thumb digit

HOW TO USE THE NUTRITION FOOD JOURNAL

For the next week enjoy the foods you eat and pay attention to how they feed your body with important nutrients.

Journal Components	Explanation	Importance
Portion Size	**Palm size** – Protein or other solid mass like pizza. **Handful size** - Carbohydrates or scatter food like beans. **The last digit of the thumb** – Fats or sweets, like butter and jelly.	Our empty stomach is the size of our fists so our hands give a reliable measurement based on our body size. Using our hands to assess portion size gives a relatively accurate measurement that requires no fancy tools or technology.
Proteins	Meats, poultry, fish, eggs, dairy, soy, beans. This group includes: the strange "meat/poultry" found in breaded nuggets from a fast food chain; hot dogs; cheese on pizza or macaroni; a bottle of milk; liquid dietary supplements; peanut butter; and yogurt products.	Proteins supply the body with essential amino acids that the body cannot make for itself. Without these amino acids our tissues break down leaving us weak, with poor resistance to disease.
Fats	Oils, cream, nuts, butter, lard, other animal fats. This group includes: margarine and other "butter substitutes"; cheese on pizza and macaroni; peanut butter; liquid dietary supplements; whole milk; whole milk cheeses; and ice cream.	Fats from animals and plants provide essential fatty acids that the body cannot make for itself. Fatty acids build the cell walls and the cells that protect our nerves (myelin). They also feed the cell components that produce energy (mitochondria).
Carbohydrates	Vegetables, fruits, grains, breads, pasta. This group includes: fruit juices; candy; cookies; crackers; "protein" bars; granola; canned spaghetti; macaroni and cheese; liquid dietary supplements; and pizza crust.	Fruits, vegetables and whole grains provide fiber, vitamins, minerals, phytonutrients and other essential micronutrients. We need these to stay healthy. Fiber keeps food moving through the GI tract and slows the absorption of sugars into the bloodstream. Beware of "added fiber" that comes from cellulose, (i.e. – sawdust).
Nutritional Quality	**Alcohol** – Wine, beer, and spirits. **Sweets** – Sugar (by any name) as one of the top three ingredients; or grams of sugar outnumber grams of protein and fat in a serving size. (Fruit juices; candy; cookies; crackers; "protein" bars; granola; liquid yogurts.) **Processed food** – Has a label with more than five ingredients, usually including one you don't immediately recognize. **Whole food** – Doesn't need a label.	**Alcohol** – Very little nutritional value. **Sugar** – Gets into the blood stream too fast and sets off mood altering responses. Provides calories without nutrients. Juices provide plenty of sugar (fructose) with none of the beneficial fiber. Fructose without fiber gets processed like alcohol in the liver – i.e. turns to fat. **Processed food** – Processed carbohydrates, white breads, crackers, puffed cereals and vegetables contain very little fiber or nutrients. Contains very few nutrients and often toxins. **Whole food** – Contains macronutrients and micronutrients in a form the body recognizes and can use.

into thirds would have similar circumference and thickness. One slice of either style of pizza would qualify as one portion. One handful of a scatter food, like salad, cereal, pasta, rice, or mixed vegetables would count as a portion size. Sweets and fats get measured by the last joint of our thumbs.

- Protein, Fat, and Carbohydrates are the three macronutrients we all need in our diets. Put a checkmark in whichever column fits. Some foods get a checkmark in more than one column. Milk contains all three macronutrients. Most meats and fish have both fat and protein.

- Nutritional Quality refers to the amount of nutrients contained in the food. Alcohol has almost no nutritional value. Sweets have calories and occasionally some minimal additional contribution to nutrition. Processed foods come with packaging that lists their ingredients and a calculated nutritional profile. Whole foods generally come as close as possible to their original state in nature. They contain the most complete nutrition as they have both components we know, as well as those we have yet to discover.

- Emotions and Sensations that come up during mealtimes or with specific foods. We all carry around a lot of emotional baggage with our food due to the attention it receives in the media and from our families and friends. Do we enjoy the food? Do we have conflicting feelings? Do we eat to soothe emotions? Jot down what comes to mind.

Exercise 4.5: Learn to Find Your Stopping Place

Registered dietician and family therapist Ellyn Satter developed an approach for treating eating disorders she calls Eating Competence (www.ellynsatterinstitute .org). Her research shows a higher correlation of positive health outcomes with Eating Competence than conventional dieting. Satter's method does not restrict what we eat, but emphasizes trusting our body's ability to choose foods that will nourish us, as we focus on how we feel physically and emotionally when eating. She teaches her clients how to recognize when they have had enough to eat (Satter, 2008):

1. If we come to our meal *famished,* we will likely eat faster and take in too much. We need to feed ourselves on a regular schedule to keep from get-

ting in that state. It's fine to feel hungry before eating, but not desperate. Three to five hours between meals works for most people, even children.

2. When does our feeling of *hunger* go away? It usually does so before we tire of the enjoyable flavors and textures.
3. When does our *appetite* leave? We'll know that point because the foods don't taste quite as good—a perfect stopping place.
4. When do we feel *full*? It's time to stop now!
5. Have we gone past *full* into feeling *stuffed*? Misery follows. A full stomach also triggers an insulin response which makes overeating particularly dangerous if we have diabetes.

Be aware of when, where, and how often we eat more than feels comfortable. Use the Emotions and Sensations column of Worksheet 4.4 to make a note of how you felt at the beginning and ending of your meal or snack. Eating too much, a feasting response, occurs for most of us after events like Thanksgiving dinner. That's okay once in a while, but not every day and at every meal.

Set an Intention and Do It: Practice Letting Go of Sugar, Flour, and Alcohol for 30 Days

The best way to release sugar, flour, and alcohol's addictive power over our eating choices involves eliminating them from our diet long enough to extinguish cravings and discover what health improvements result. Although we may anticipate difficulty with eliminating these three foods, my clients tell me this practice is the easiest of all I recommend.

We get multiple opportunities to follow this practice every day. Our goal of 90% means an occasional slip doesn't signal a failure. When we add in our three friends—fat, fiber, and fermented foods (those with natural probiotics), we find that cravings go away in a matter of days.

Focus on all the great foods we can eat. If we've been avoiding nuts, cream, butter, steak and other high-fat foods by following outdated low-fat recommendations, we can enjoy reintroducing them. They reduce hunger cravings between meals and are harder to overeat because they trigger all our neurohormonal feedback loops that tell us we have eaten enough (Lustig, 2013).

Exercise 4.6: Set an Intention to Connect with Earth Energy

Before eating, we can take a moment to put one hand over our upper abdomen, above the belly button, and another on our lower abdomen below the belly button. With eyes closed, spend few seconds to take in the miracle of digestion. We can forgive ourselves any eating transgressions we may have committed. Our stomach and the rest of our digestive system have already taken care of them. Let our friends (our guts and the microorganisms who make them home) know we plan to work *with* them during this meal.

Take it meal by meal and day by day. Explore new foods and enjoy old favorites. Pay attention to that feeling of satisfaction. Pay attention to energy, sleep, moods, and health conditions. Most people see almost immediate improvements in some or all of these within days. After a month of no sugar, no flour, no alcohol, we may see even more changes for the better.

Exercise 4.7: Enjoy Detoxing for a Month with Foods You Love

During this practice we cleanse our bodies of the big three addictive toxins, SUGAR, FLOUR, and ALCOHOL. We can use our three friends, FAT, FIBER, and FERMENTED FOODS to help us get over these addictions and cravings by building our body's strength and resilience. These friendly foods have an asterisk next to them.

We give ourselves the gift of success by not letting perfection be the enemy of good: 90% is great; 80% is good. If we slip up—no worries—keep going. Pay attention to how eating feels. Get enough!

Eat what you love! Love what you eat!

Foods to Enjoy	Foods to Avoid
Beef	Fried Meats
Pork	Breaded Meats
Lamb	Sweet Sauces
Chicken	Gravies Made With Flour
*Hamburger	
*Sausage	
Fish	Fried Fish
Shellfish	Breaded Fish
Tofu	Sweet Sauces Added
*Miso	
*Tempeh	
*Vegetables, Fresh	
*Vegetables, Frozen	Sweet Sauces Added
*Vegetables, Canned	Canned With Sugar Added
*Fruits, Fresh	Fruit Juices
*Fruits, Frozen	Frozen With Sugar Added
Fruits, Canned	Canned In Syrup
*Bulgar/Cracked Wheat	Whole Wheat Or White Bread
*Steel-Cut Oats	Oat Flour Or Bread
*Corn Or Hominy	Corn Meal, Tortillas, Chips
*Rye Grains	Rye Bread Or Crackers
*Quinoa	Quinoa Chips Or Crackers
*Brown Rice	Rice Cakes
White Rice	Rice Crackers
Milk, Whole	Flavored Milks
Half And Half	Low-Fat Half And Half
*Cream	Ice Cream, Cool Whip
Cream Cheese	Low-Fat Cream Cheese
*Butter	Margarine
*Sour Cream	Low-Fat Sour Cream
Yogurt, Whole Milk	Low-Fat Yogurt

* Friendly foods

Make It Ours: Practice Eating for Health Transformation

Learn to make delicious desserts without sugar and flour. Find delightful beverages that have no sugar or alcohol. As sugar, flour, and alcohol leave our bodies, we discover that we can taste other flavors better. Experiment with spices and herbs. These flavorful plant materials carry important micronutrients that help us stay healthy and make our foods taste better (Katzen & Edelson, 2015).

Once we have stayed on the no-sugar, no-flour, no-alcohol practice for a month we can begin to think about extending this practice or modifying it to suit our personal health concerns. Most people see improvements in thinking, mood, energy, and other health markers after a month. We have calmed down the inflammation in our bodies caused by toxic reactions to sugar, flour, and alcohol. Now, we can proceed in several ways.

Exercise 4.8: Exploring Food with the Food and Mood Journal

Some of us have had improvements but want to check what happens with further elimination of potential "trigger foods", those foods that may trigger symptoms such as the following common food-related health issues:

Ears   otitis media (ear infections)

Nose   nasal congestion, sneezing, runny nose

Eyes   tearing, puffy eyes, dark circles under eyes

Oral   swelling of lips, tongue, mouth, & throat

Skin   hives, eczema, red cheeks, itching

Respiratory   difficulty breathing, cough, wheezing, asthma

Intestinal   reflux, vomiting, nausea, abdominal pain, diarrhea, constipation

Neurological   headache, migraine, and behaviors such as emotional outbursts, irritability, and hyperactivity. (Strickland, 2009)

Many people restrict eggs, dairy, nightshades (tomatoes, potatoes, eggplants, peppers), grains of all kinds, or legumes (beans). Instead of eliminating all of them at once, try one category at a time for a week or 10 days and see what happens. Then eat some of that food. If we have a sensitivity to that food we usually notice it immediately after a week of avoiding it. Generally, once sugar, flour, and alcohol have been eliminated we can see pretty immediate results with these other groups. Experiment with cutting back on these other foods and explore the results.

Some of us feel happy with the changes we have seen and want to see what happens if we eat sugar, flour, or alcohol on an occasional basis, at parties or other special occasions. Instead of reintroducing them all at once, try one during meals or snacks for a few days. Watch to see what happens. We may see symptoms pop up that we never associated with these foods. Our bodies have calmed down the inflammatory processes associated with sugar, flour, and alcohol just enough for our immune systems to take a break. Because sensitivities still exist, our immune systems will very quickly mount a response. Sometimes our bodies respond to the reintroduction of sugar, flour, or alcohol within minutes, but more often it takes hours to notice a response. Use Worksheet 4.8: The Food and Mood Journal to track responses to sugar, flour, and alcohol as you reintroduce them as well as with any other foods that you would like to explore as potential "trigger foods".

Bringing sugar, flour, alcohol, or other "trigger" foods back into our diet becomes an individual choice. I often recommend reintroducing a favorite after giving our bodies a few months or even years to heal. I usually never say never to specific foods because we need variety in our diets to stay healthy. Our reactions to food change over time, and variety keeps our gut microbes happy and immune systems exercised. Schedule sugar, flour, alcohol, and beloved "trigger" foods for special times and places. That helps us enjoy them without letting them create chronic health issues.

Share It: Fasting and Feasting with Friends and Family

Sugar, flour, and alcohol have inherently addicting qualities. Once we eat a little, we invariably want more. They can creep up on us and soon we find ourselves back in old eating patterns again. One way to combat this tendency is to schedule regular periods of "detoxing" through fasting.

Every spiritual tradition has ritualized periods of fasting. Many of these occur seasonally. Some we observe weekly, and others mark rites of passage at vari-

Worksheet 4.8: Food and Mood Journal

Name:_____   **Start Date:** _____   **Finish Date:** _____

Use this form to look for food sensitivities. Avoid a particular food for a week to 10 days, then eat a lot of it for the next few days. Use the numbers for Enjoyment, Feelings, and Behavior to make this easier and quicker. Jot down any other symptoms from the symptom list on the next page. Take a minimum of 2 hours between each meal or snack to give the body time to regulate blood sugar and to get a more accurate accounting of reactions to foods. Chart these reactions prior to the next meal or snack in the 2 Hours + column.

Date	Foods Eaten Meals or Snacks	Immediate Enjoyment / Behavior	30 Min Later Feelings / Behavior	2 Hours + Feelings / Behavior

Immediate Enjoyment: 5 = Delicious – the best food ever / 1 = Yuck – I never want to see it again
Feelings: 5 = Feeling Fine – happy & full of energy / 1 = Hungry, headaches, shaky & grouchy
Behavior: 5 = Calm, content, focused / 1 = Hyperactive, irritable, distractible, emotional outbursts

ous times in our lives. Use these opportunities when they happen in your spiritual community. Giving up sugar, flour, and alcohol with a larger group makes it easier. We can use these times to remind ourselves to go easy or eliminate sugar, flour, and alcohol.

We can create our own rituals. Many people do intermittent fasts, where they do not eat for 12 to 16 hours daily. These fasting periods generally have special meals and foods associated with ending the mini-fast. We even have a name for some of them: breakfast! Perhaps we want to try intermittent fasting in our own life.

Longer term fasting for 3 to 5 days may provide even more benefits. In the absence of sufficient nutrients, our bodies begin to scavenge damaged and diseased cells. Then our bodies activate stem cells to replace these diseased cells with brand new, healthy ones. Valter Longo, a cell biologist and director of the Longevity Center at the University of Southern California, has researched these phenomena for decades and written a book, *The Longevity Diet,* which explains his studies and offers suggestions for the interested nonscientist.

We can develop "signature" dishes with traditional preparations, fermented foods, and beverages. Work on finding recipes that get compliments, even when they contain little or no sugar, flour, or alcohol. I like to bake, and I have a sweet tooth, but I've learned that I can take almost any recipe and use half as much sugar as recommended. Most people rave about the results. When there is less sugar in the mix, they can taste the butter and eggs.

I also have a few favorite recipes that use traditional soaking preparations for whole grain flour in baked goods. Soaking eliminates the bitterness of whole grain flour, which has more fiber and protein than white flour. I have memorized my favorite recipes through repeated use. These have become my signature dishes, the special occasion foods that I bring to potlucks and family dinners. It's always a thrill, and a rush of serotonin, to see them disappear in a hurry. Develop your own.

Eat what you love. Love what you eat.

Exercise 4.9: Eating with Children

Just as adults have trouble with sugar and flour addictions, so do children. "Kid's Menus" and other supposedly child-friendly foods all contain significant quantities of sugar, with toxic fructose levels (Lustig, 2013). We see this in the increasing numbers of children diagnosed with obesity, type 2 diabetes, and nonalcoholic fatty liver disease. Many families experience picky eating challenges with children, who choose starchy, sweet foods over all others. Food allergies, food sensitivities, hyperactivity, and moodiness all share some relationship to the blood glucose roller coaster produced by the large quantity of sugars and flours children eat.

Even more than adults, children need a large percentage of dietary fats and protein in order to grow their bodies. Bones, brains, muscles, and hormones especially benefit from high-fat and high-protein diets. Historically, most pre-industrial cultures made sure children, pregnant women, and nursing mothers got these foods, even when they were otherwise in short supply.

Food anxiety translates into mealtime battles with children, especially over vegetables which, while important, take a back seat, nutritionally speaking, to fat and protein. According to Ellyn Satter, a registered dietician and psychotherapist, mealtime battles, negotiations, and bargaining never provide an answer. Instead she recommends a division of responsibility in feeding.

In summary, Satter says:

- Adults must choose *what* to serve, *when* to serve meals on a schedule, *where* to eat those meals or snacks (at the table), and *how* to behave during mealtimes.
- Do not respond (positively or negatively) to a child's food choices or refusals. We cannot know what our children feel, smell, or taste. Eating is always entirely self-regulated, so children must explore foods on their own terms.

Before putting ourselves and our families on a no-sugar, no-flour diet, we need to first expand their food choices to include offerings that reduce or eliminate flour and sugar. If we live with a picky eater, we may need to first establish Satter's division of responsibility in feeding.

1. *Teach by example.* Make one meal that everyone shares. Stop short-order cooking individual dishes. Include at least one dish that a child willingly eats. Generally, this will be bread, rice, pasta, or small animal-shaped crackers. That's okay. Use this food as a side dish. Otherwise, cook foods the rest of the family likes. Let children pick and choose what to explore.

2. *Teach table manners, not nutrition.* Children can learn the following two responses to a food offering:

   "Yes, please."

   "No, thank you."

   These are polite responses. "Yuck" is not a polite word at mealtimes, because it hurts the cook's feelings. (Life might improve for all of us if adults learned to use these polite responses instead of endlessly explaining their medical conditions and philosophical beliefs about food.)

3. *Stop arguing or giving nutritional lectures at mealtimes.* Let children pick and choose what to explore, what to eat, and what to refuse. Numerous studies show that children will spontaneously balance their diets when given a variety of nutritious foods. Each mealtime does not have to include all three macronutrients. Once sugar becomes a sometimes food and not an everyday food, children will balance their nutritional needs over days, weeks, and months, rarely at the same meal.

   When children refuse food, the following three phrases will magically end food fights and make mealtimes more pleasant:

   "You don't have to eat that" (Anderson, 2015)

   "Good. That leaves more for the rest of us" (my mother's favorite line!)

   "That's okay. You just haven't tasted it enough times yet. You'll like it when you grow up." (Le Billion, 2014)

4. *Serve meals at regularly scheduled times, with no snacks between meals.* We all eat better when we come to the table a little hungry.

5. *Stop serving any store-bought sweets at home.* Sugar addiction is no joke. Food manufacturers spend billions of dollars developing marketing strategies known in the industry as the "nag factor." Food shopping with a child will instantly alert us to the foods that have successfully employed this strategy for getting adults to buy costly, but rarely nutritious, foods (Ludwig, 2007).

Make all desserts at home. Serve sweet, ripe, fresh fruits often. When baking, reduce the sugar content by half. Follow recipes that include eggs, butter, and milk. These ingredients make desserts nutritious as well as delicious. Then, if dessert is all our children eat, at least we know they got some nutritional benefit eating it. Serve desserts in single serving sizes, with a "no seconds" policy. If children refuse to eat a homemade dessert because they have a brand loyalty, then our "Good, more for the rest of us," has more meaning. Children who watch their siblings and parents carefully carve up their refused dessert portion soon begin trying these coveted treats.

Putting vegetables into desserts works fine, as long as we don't sneak them in, which adversely affects trust in parent-child relationships. Let children know they are eating vegetables in a dessert and they may be more willing to explore that vegetable later in a different presentation.

Enjoy mealtimes with your children. Teach them to eat what they love and love what they eat.

Exercise 4.10: Eating with Elders

Our senses of smell, taste, and touch can deteriorate as we age. Shopping and preparing food often becomes a neglected chore, especially when there is no one around to share that meal. Like children, elders fall prey to convenience foods with higher than average sugar-and-flour content.

To maintain the health of bones, brains, and body, elders, like children, benefit from a high-fat, high-protein diet. Elders, like young children, eat smaller portions of food; therefore, we want to pack a lot of nutrition into a small package (fats fit this bill nicely).

Elders don't have a lifetime in front of them, as children do, but we still need to enjoy our meals and we always do that better when we can share them with others. Shared meals have emotional nourishment as well as nutrition.

Sometimes elders have some difficulty with chewing and swallowing, so often their foods get chopped up and blended. Soups and casseroles work perfectly for making delicious and nutritious easy-eating options, but remember to prepare dishes that look good and taste good. Soup and casserole cookbooks abound, and these easy-eating options also work well for children and adults with or without chewing and swallowing challenges.

Lectures, arguing, negotiating, and bargaining about food choices have even less success with elders than they do with children. Lifetime patterns of eating will be difficult or impossible to change.

Eventually, a time may come when elders can no longer bring a spoon to their mouth. We must remember to have patience when this time comes. As much as we want to encourage their independence we might have to accept a new level of care. A client once asked me how to feed her ailing father. "Like a lover," I replied.

In all times and all ages it boils down to:

Eat what you love. Love what you eat.

CHAPTER 5

Metal Energies

Learn! Find Inspiration in Work

Man, through the use of his hands, as they are energized
by mind and will, can influence the state of his own health.

—MARY REILLY

METAL ATTRACTS US. Stardust, gold, copper, silver, tin, iron, mercury, and diamonds have captivated human imagination since before any of us can remember. Currencies of gods and mortals, metals have deep mythic associations and value beyond their beauty and function.

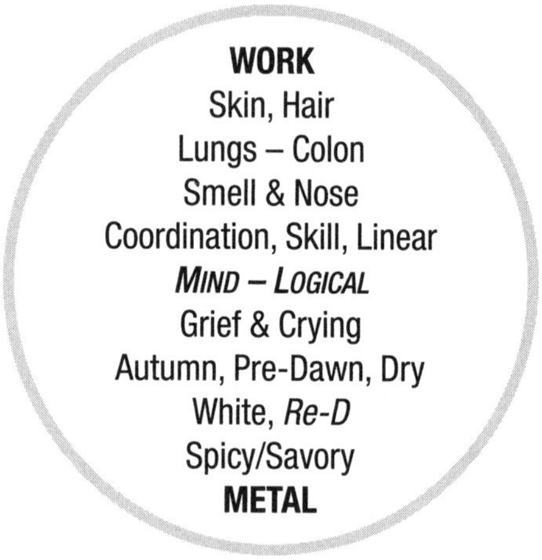

Genies, leprechauns, trolls, dactyls, dragons, and goblins have legendary associations with mining, metalworking, and hoarding treasure. Their often diminished, ugly appearance and sharp teeth might serve as allegory to what happens

WORK
Skin, Hair
Lungs – Colon
Smell & Nose
Coordination, Skill, Linear
Mind – Logical
Grief & Crying
Autumn, Pre-Dawn, Dry
White, *Re-D*
Spicy/Savory
METAL

Figure 5.1 Life Aspects Associated with Metal Energies

when greed for material riches gets the upper hand. King Midas, who prayed for the gift to turn everything he touched to gold, first destroyed his daughter by turning her into a gold statue, and then starved as everything he touched turned to inedible gold. Lessons such as these find their way into stories from many cultures.

Diamond-hard dactyls, from Greek legend, sprung from the ground as the Earth Mother dug her fingers into the dirt while giving birth to the gods. These

10 indestructible chthonic spirit-men, who gave their name to our 10 fingers, taught healing and metalworking to mortals. Our human ability to imagine an outcome and create that outcome through the work of our hands and mind has led us to great beauty as well as our own destruction.

Humans use metals for tools and adornment. We began saving useful rocks and shiny treasures millions of years ago. Over time, we started shaping these Metals to suit our needs and fancies. First we chipped rocks into all manner of tools. Then about six thousand years ago we found that gold, copper, silver, lead, tin, and iron responded well to heat, and we figured out how to fashion intricate and elaborate adornments and more varied and specialized tools.

Metals appear in predictably organized molecular structures, held together by strong bonds. Mendeleev dreamed up the Periodic Table that gives a numerical value, based on that element's molecular weight, to each element we have found in our universe. Scientists divide them into metals, metalloids, and nonmetals, but in this book we will consider every one of these timeless startdust-elements Metal. (Matthew, 2016)

A billion years ago, carbon, a nonmetal and the molecular basis of life on earth, became diamonds under heat and pressure 100 miles deep in the earth. Lava brought those diamonds to the surface where we could find them. Diamonds, the only single-element gemstone and the hardest naturally occurring substance on the planet, are made of carbon atoms bonded together in groups of five. Together they form a network, a crystalline structure, with bonds so strong that each crystal forms a giant molecule.

Archaeologists measure time through the dominant metal-based technologies used during that era. Stone tools from more than three million years ago predate our origins as Homo sapiens, or very likely even our genus Homo.. Stone tools became increasingly more specialized, allowing for farming, building, pottery, and working soft metals such as gold, copper, and silver some ten to sixty thousand years ago. Spinning, weaving, sewing, making music, writing, rowing, wheels, domesticating animals, and fermenting of alcohol began during the Paleolithic and Neolithic eras. Stonehenge was built at the end of this era.

As tens of thousands of years went by, humans became more proficient at using fire to smelt metals found in rock. The soft metals, gold, copper, silver, and lead, did not hold an edge like rock, but copper mixed with tin produced bronze, and another era of Metal technology evolved. Bronze Age advancements in technology included swords, sailing, musical notation, money, more forms of writing, and the making of paper from papyrus. Bronze tools persisted for many thousands of years in different areas of the world, but in the cultures surrounding the Mediterranean, this era ended about three thousand years ago (1200 BC) with the destruction of most of its cities through warfare and natural disasters. Egypt, under Ramses III, fared the best, with Memphis, Tyre, Sais, and Tanis (where Moses is supposed to have been found in the reeds) all surviving the collapse of the Mediterranean Bronze Age civilization. Babylon, a Bronze Age city state in what is now Iraq, along with three cities from the Assyrian Empire, and Sardis in the Hittite Empire all survived until later eras. The loss of extensive international trade between those nations led to the dark age that followed the collapse of the Bronze Age which resulted in the loss of many arts and technologies (Cline, 2014).

Iron-based tools and technologies rose from the ruins at the end of the Bronze Age. People created glass, false teeth, lighthouses, cranks, cranes, crossbows, catapults, warships, fishing reels, woodblock printing, stirrups, horse collars, arched bridges, and paddle-wheel boats. In the first century A.D. Hero of Alexandria developed a heat operated automatic door, a coin-operated vending machine to dispense holy water, and the undoubtedly popular and not yet replicated bottomless wine glass (Jaffe, 2006). The Iron Age took those of us in

H 1 *B*																	He 2 *B*
Li 3 *C*	Be 4 *C*											B 5 *C*	C 6 *SN/L*	N 7 *SN/L*	O 8 *SN/L*	F 9 *L*	Ne 10 *SN/L*
Na 11 *L*	Mg 12 *L*											Al 13 *SN/L*	Si 14 *SN/L*	P 15 *SN/L*	S 16 *SN/L*	Cl 17 *L*	Ar 18 *L*
K 19 *L*	Ca 20 *L*	Sc 21 *L*	Ti 22 *SN/L*	V 23 *SN/L*	Cr 24 *L*	Mn 25 *L*	Fe 26 *SN/L*	Co 27 *SN*	Ni 28 *SN/*	Cu 29 *L*	Zn 30 *L*	Ga 31 *SN*	Ge 32 *SN*	As 33 *L*	Se 34 *SN*	Br 35 *SN*	Kr 36 *SN*
Rb 37 *SN*	Sr 38 *L*	Y 39 *L*	Zr 40 *L*	Nb 41 *L*	Mo 42 *SN/L*	Tc 43 *L*	Ru 44 *SN/L*	Rh 45 *SN*	Pd 46 *SN/L*	Ag 47 *SN/L*	Cd 48 *SN/L*	In 49 *SN/L*	Sn 50 *SN*	Sb 51 *SN*	Te 52 *SB*	I 53 *SN*	Xe 54 *SN*
Cs 55 *SN*	Ba 56 *L*		Hf 72 *SN/L*	Ta 73 *SN/L*	W 74 *SN/L*	Re 75 *SN*	Os 76 *SN*	Ir 77 *SN*	Pt 78 *SN*	Au 79 *SN*	Hg 80 *SN/L*	Tl 81 *SN/L*	Pb 82 *SN*	Bi 83 *SN*	Po 84 *SN*	At 85 *SN*	Rn 86 *SN*
Fr 87 *SN*	Ra 88 *SN*																

La 57 *L*	Ce 58 *L*	Pr 59 *SN/L*	Nd 60 *SN/L*	Pm 61 *SN/L*	Sm 62 *SN/L*	Eu 63 *SN*	Gd 64 *SN*	Tb 65 *SN*	Dy 66 *SN*	Ho 67 *SN*	Er 68 *SN*	Tm 69 *SN*	Yb 70 *SN/L*	Lu 71 *SN*
Ac 89 *SN*	Th 90 *SN*	Pa 91 *SN*	U 92 *SN*	Np 93 *SN*	Pu 94 *SN*	Am 95 *M*	Cm 96 *M*	Bk 97 *M*	Cf 98 *M*	Es 99 *M*	Fm 100 *M*	Md 101 *M*	No 102 *M*	Lr 103 *M*

Figure 5.2 The Contemporary Periodic Table of Elements. The original table from Mendeleev had only 63 shaded elements, but his basic organization accommodated the discovery of new elements. The italics indicate the origin of the elements as follows   B=Big Bang; C=Cosmic rays; L=Large stars; S=Small stars; SN=Supernovae; M=Man-made. (Matthew, 2016)

Western civilization from the collapse of the Bronze Age civilizations to the collapse of the Roman Empire at the beginning of the Middle Ages.

Knowledge, technology, art, music, and writing have shaped human destiny from long before we can remember. The worlds we have created and destroyed through what we make with minds and hands resonate with Metal energy. We work every day, learn from our mistakes, grieve any losses that accompany such learning, and go on doing whatever we need to do to create comfort, safety, and beauty for ourselves and our communities.

Exercise 5.1: Making a Conscious Connection to Metal Energy

Go out and look at the night sky. Are the moon or any stars visible? The moon is generally visible as it swells from crescent to full, then it rises so late we may be asleep and sets during the day. Sometimes we can see the moon as it shrinks from full back to crescent during the daytime. Planets appear as bright stars. They move around the night sky in unique trajectories that take them through various constellations. Astrologers and astronomers have studied and charted

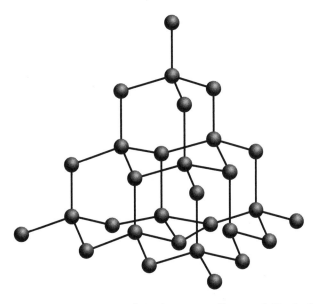

Figure 5.3 The molecular structure of Carbon as a diamond. Each ring of five Carbon atoms connects to another ring, forming a single molecule of Carbon.

these movements for thousands of years. Take a look at a star chart, or check out a phone application and try to identify the stars on the chart or screen. Imagine the days when people measured time by changes in the night sky. How much learning and practice would we need to do that?

Practice Eliminating Clutter: Prepare for Inspiration

Our habit for this element involves elimination of clutter to give us more breathing room—a blanker canvas that invites inspiration. We live in an economy that depends on constant consumption of disposable items. This means almost every one of us has more than we need or even want. The stuff we keep "in case we need it" collects on surfaces, as well as in corners, cupboards, closets, garages, attics, basements, and expensive storage facilities.

For millions of years we depended on stashes of food, tools, fibers, and building materials, but those days are long past. Now our collections serve as refuge for whole colonies of bacteria, viruses, dust mites, and even larger, more visible and disturbing wildlife. They no longer serve our survival; in fact, they shorten our lives by reducing the quality of the air we breathe and increasing the stress of "unfinished business"—whether that business is cleaning, fixing, returning something borrowed, or completing a project.

Books on decluttering abound. I've read lots of rules and systems, and they all work—if you do them. By far the simplest guideline I've found came from Karen Kingston's *Creating Sacred Space with Feng Shui: Learn the Art of Space Clearing and Bring New Energy into Your Life:*

>   *If you don't love an object, let it go.*

When Kingston says "love" she means something that brings intrinsic joy through its beauty, usefulness, or both. Most of us hold onto many objects because they remind us of important people, or significant events, even if we don't necessarily enjoy the object on its own merits.

Letting go of these objects activates an emotional response, frequently grief for what the object represents: a loved one, happy times, missed opportunity, or well-spent youth. Avoiding sadness leads to clutter. Shedding tears of grief (and maybe even relief) as we let them go heals the body, whereas holding on to them is far more likely to result in tears we shed from allergies. Learning to grieve, like learning anything, takes repetition and practice. Life will provide us with plenty of opportunities to grieve.

Our habit for this chapter addresses the practice of decluttering by quantifying the amount of time or the number of objects we let go every day to a multiple of 5.

We can spend 5 to 15 minutes of each day letting go of what we do not need. Or we can get rid of the first 5 to 15 things we no longer need every day. Junk mail, magazines, trash, uneaten food, clothes that don't fit, furniture no one uses, toys from children who have moved away, school memorabilia, cards, letters, and photos all make great choices. These can go to the garbage can, recycling bin, charity, or back to the person who loaned it to us. Do not spend a lot of thought on where to put this waste. Get it out of the house and out of the car today. We need to make decluttering a daily habit like brushing our teeth or sitting on the porcelain throne.

A real "get rid of weight fast" diet makes use of weighing the stuff before we get rid of it! And by the way, decluttering often leads to bodily weight reduction as well. Another of my favorite decluttering book titles comes from Peter Walsh, *Does This Clutter Make My Butt Look Fat? An Easy Plan for Losing Weight and Living More.* Walsh makes some very direct links between the clutter in our homes and the clutter on our bodies and shows how getting rid of stuff aids us in weight loss as well.

Practice, Practice, Practice: Developing Skills

"Work" has joined the ranks of four-letter curses. On our Healing Compass, Work sits opposite Play on a continuum which we usually think of as "fun" and "not so fun," and yet we did not always hold Work in such low regard.

We have always needed to get food, water, and shelter to survive. Many of us grow vegetables, raise animals, fish, hunt, and build for "fun," although few of us depend exclusively on our own manual labor to secure food, water, and shelter. We have become dependent on a global system of corporations and industries that supply them to us in exchange for money. Most of us work for money to buy everything we want, need, and hopefully can afford.

No so long ago we had no separation from work and home. Our days began with sunrise and ended soon after sunset. We made everything we used, or traded with neighbors who had skills we lacked. In *Ascent of Humanity:*

Civilization and the Human Sense of Self, Charles Eisenstein discusses the role that assembly-line manufacturing played in developing low-skill or single-skill jobs, the very jobs increasingly given to robots today. Before automobile assembly lines, carriage builders made the entire auto body, but they worked too slowly and carefully. The automobiles lasted too long and cost too much. Assembly-line manufacturing made it possible to sell more cars for less money and greater corporate profits. It also served to fill our landscape and landfills with discarded vehicles, and their heavy metal batteries.

Matthew Crawford explores the theme of meaningful work in the lives of white-collar cubicle workers and even bankers whose jobs have become increasingly rote. *Shop Class as Soul Craft: An Inquiry into the Value of Work*, chronicles his journey from electrician, to PhD, to motorcycle repair person. His transition from electrician to "knowledge worker" involved getting a master's degree and resulted in both mind-numbing work days and a lower annual income.

Crawford explains that his jobs as an electrician and motorcycle mechanic both involved analyzing varied and often complex problems, arriving at a solution, and testing his ideas by completing the project. He enjoyed his academic studies for much the same reason. His white-collar job involved skimming through technical and scientific articles and summarizing them into a few sentences, which quickly grew rote and uninteresting. This entry-level publishing job paid much less than his electrical work had.

In *The Continuum Concept: In Search of Happiness Lost*, Jean Leidoff describes living with a group of self-sufficient people in the South American jungle. She watches them laugh at the bumps, scrapes, and bruises they get carrying a heavy dugout canoe over a difficult portage, while the Europeans travelling with her suffer similar bumps, scrapes, and bruises, which leads them to curse rather than laugh at their plight. She struggles carrying water up the steep river banks and imagines a system of pulleys and ropes that would make the job easier, until she notices that the women take great pride in their ability to carry water up the slope without spilling a drop—something they have practiced since childhood and at which they have great skill.

We all need work that stimulates our happy hormones. We get dopamine whenever we set a goal or a quota and meet it. We get dopamine when we check off items on our "to do" lists and when we complete a project. Ideally, most jobs involve some or all of these kinds of tasks, although dopamine bursts wane quickly without variety in the tasks at hand.

Our bursts of serotonin come from recognition. We get those bursts whenever we have other people to "boss" around. We also get it when people recognize a job well done.

Endorphins generally come most frequently to those who do heavy manual labor. Any time we work muscles to the point of microtearing muscle fibers, our bodies release endorphins. We could think of this as a "laborer's high" similar to the "runners high." Farmers, construction workers, and others who do similar jobs may experience this, and like athletes, sometimes injury as well.

We get oxytocin bursts from enjoying our colleagues and people who come to us for services rendered, regardless of the amount of physical labor required by our work. The two South American men having fun on the difficult portage had plenty of oxytocin to keep them laughing. The European men had very little, in spite of their close proximity under the heavy canoe. What was the difference?

Perhaps, each group had a different narrative about their jobs. The South American men may have seen the portage as a challenge, a game of endurance they could share. The European men, like Jean Leidoff carrying water up the hill, saw it as drudgery, something that could have been eased if only they had a road or some other more modern form of assistance. So the South Americans found humor in their foibles, where the Europeans grieved their hardships, wishing for an easier portage they could not have.

If we understand that we can choose actions and perspectives that make our happy hormones flow, we might use this knowledge to tune in to our work and mine it for pleasure instead of pain. Setting daily goals, recognizing the value of our own efforts, and finding colleagues to share our challenges and victories all help to keep the happy hormones in play.

The repetitive nature of work provides a medium for learning through practice. Those of us with a gift for doing something well only enhance that gift through repetitive practice, but even a rote job can involve a kind of mindfulness meditation type of practice. Learning a skill produces happy hormones when we succeed at meeting or exceeding a new level of skill or have someone else recognize our progress. These hormones drive us to practice because we enjoy the accompanying bursts of dopamine and serotonin. These hormones dissipate quickly and so we benefit from frequent opportunities to trigger them again. In effect, we're hardwired to become accomplished in manual, cognitive, and even spiritual skills.

How do we learn a skill? We often talk about muscle memory. Although our muscles play a role in determining and remembering how much muscle force we need to produce a desired action, our movements actually get coordinated from "skin memory" (Greene & Roberts, 2017). Our skin is filled with all kinds of specialized nerve endings that can sense pressure, stretch, location, temperature, and pain. These sensors convey a dizzying array of information to our spinal cords, brain stem, cerebellum, limbic system, and cortex.

The spinal cord processes pain and temperature immediately to prevent damage to tissues. It also sends information to the brain for processing in various areas, notably a strip of brain tissue called the sensory strip. The sensory strip communicates with the motor strip, with multiple side trips to various parts of the limbic system coordinating other senses, most especially vision and hearing. Other parts of the brain get involved as well. When all that information gets sorted out, in nanoseconds, information travels to the motor strip, and the correct movements get underway via the cerebellum, limbic system, and brain stem.

With repetition and practice our skin, muscles, and brain work together to coordinate movement. The neurons responsible for this complex network of connections get established during sleep before and after birth, with most of them completed in our first year of life, constructed from fatty acids in our mother's milk. Activities that catch our interest during the first few years of life engage us in repetitive practice that strengthens specific neural pathways and sets our course to develop the roles we will assume as adults.

We can learn new movement patterns at any age, but for the first few years of life motor learning seems almost effortless. *In Respect the Spindle,* Abby Franquemont recounts accompanying her parents on their Peace Corps trip to the Peruvian Andes. Although only 5 years old at the time, she was several years behind the other children who had been spinning threads as part of their daily play since they could walk. One of the children's favorite games involved standing on Incan ruins and dropping their spindles over the wall, then retrieving them with the strong threads they had spun. Abby spent a lot of time running down the hill to retrieve her spindle when her threads broke. By age eight, she had mastered passable quality thread, but she never achieved the speed with which her same-age peers produced similar yardage. When she returned to the United States at age eight, her ability to turn fiber into thread with a drop spindle surpassed most of the adult spinners she met.

Lest we scoff at the ability to produce thread from a child's top, make note that this Stone Age tool produced all the threads used in European sails on ships that circumnavigated the globe during centuries of exploration and colonization. Spinning wheels made their appearance in Europe from the 13th century onward, but they couldn't spin the quality of threads needed for tough sailing cloth until the beginning of the 19th century (Franquemont, 2009).

We repeat what we most enjoy doing. As the old joke goes, a tourist asks, "How do I get to Carnegie Hall?" And a New Yorker replies, "Practice, practice, practice." All skilled movements require practice, whether we are surgeons, mechanics, athletes, artists, musicians, or housekeepers. In the beginning it may seem like play, but over time we repeat it to get the dopamine rush of succeeding at some challenging detail or the serotonin and oxytocin rush of acclaim from our peers.

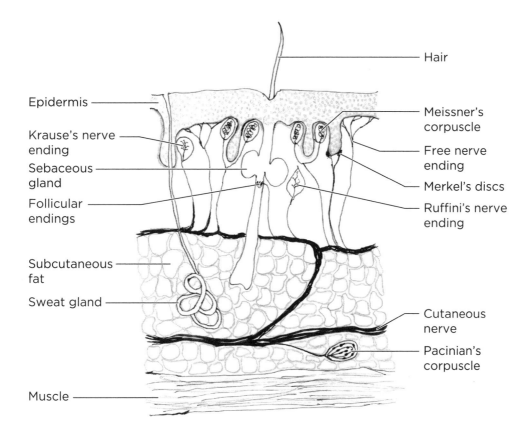

Figure 5.4 Sensory Organs Found in the Skin. Free nerve endings sense pain. Ruffini's and Krause endings sense temperature. Pacinian and Meissner's corpuscles as well as Merkel's disks sense various kinds of pressure and other touch. As skin stretches over joints all of these endings get activated and send energetic messages to the brain for analysis and response. Skin sensory organs along with sensory organs from tendons, joints, and muscles play a large role in how we regulate and coordinate movement.

We also need to practice some basic skills just to get by. An ancient story from Asia involves the monk who asks his master, "What will I do before I reach enlightenment?" The master tells him, "Chop wood and carry water." "And what will I do after enlightenment?" he continues. The master replies, "Chop wood and carry water." Our lives are filled with these moments of doing what needs to be done, whether we enjoy it or not. When we can take pride in success, or joy in the experience, life has more meaning for us. We can change our story, and doing so also takes practice.

Exercise 5.2: Conduct a Sensory-Motor Experiment

To get a sense of how these complex sensory-motor communication pathways work, we take a bath. Adjust the hot water so that it comes out of the tap in single drops. Get it as hot as possible. Lie back and put the tip of one big toe under the faucet. Because the sensory nerve from our toe to our spinal cord is

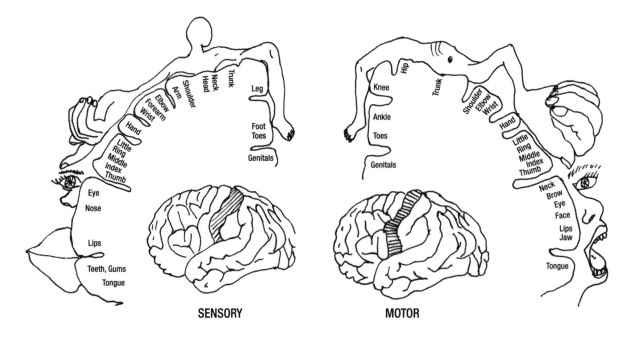

Figure 5.5 Sensory motor homunculus in the cortex, showing the relative amounts of neural tissue devoted to body sensations and movement. The size of the body parts drawn along the outer rim of the cortex show which body parts have the most neurons devoted to sensation or movement. Their location indicates where in the cortex we generally find these neurons.

the longest nerve in our body we will see the drop hit our toe before we feel it. If the water is hot enough we will automatically pull our foot away from the water, even before we sense it touching our toe, but not before seeing it.

Generally speaking, a level of heat that would damage skin tissue if we submerged our toes in it will not run out of our home plumbing for obvious safety reasons, so we may not get the automatic withdrawal response. The thoughts we think during the experiment will also affect our movement, and even sensation. If we worry about getting burned, we may pull away as we see the drop, before it registers as either touch or pain. With the exception of pulling our toe away from a painfully hot drop of water (which takes only two neurons) all of these other reactions take many more neurons than we have room to list in this box. All those connections slow down response time, but we can usually see and then feel the drop in less than a second.

Mind Over Matter: Letting Go of Our Attachments to Stuff

Beliefs create thoughts.
Thoughts create emotions.
Emotions create actions.
Actions create health.

If we *believe* that our work only has meaning when measured in monetary rewards we may *focus* on numbers and all the things that money can buy. Like Sam Polk, author of *For the Love of Money: A Memoir*, we may find ourselves *angry* and *envious* when we only get a bonus of a million and a half dollars if someone else gets more (Polk, 2014). Caught up in this endless cortisol-serotonin loop, we become willing to trade off both health and relationships as we strive to achieve more and more money.

If we *believe* our work has intrinsic meaning we can *focus* on developing skills, creating relationships within our communities, and staying healthy to enjoy our good fortune. Like Lobsang Samden, elder brother of the Dalai Lama, we can find *satisfaction* while working as a janitor in a New Jersey high school, without regretting past honors serving as a Tibetan emissary to China or the high political and religious status of his siblings (Kaplan, 1976). We can enjoy our day-to-day accomplishments, take pleasure in our family and friends, and feel healing gratitude for what we have rather than mourning what we don't.

Not all skills require the use of our hands. Daniel Goleman and Richard Davidson, authors of *Altered Traits: Science Reveals How Meditation Changes Your Mind, Brain, and Body*, began studying the neurological effects of meditation in the 1970s. They made it a part of their academic as well as personal practice. They have watched and analyzed the brains of people who have just learned to meditate and Tibetan monks with as much as 60,000 hours of practice.

That's a lot of time. Consider this: If we spend an hour a day meditating, at the end of a year we will have logged about 350 hours. (That gives us roughly a two-week vacation from practice.) By the end of 3 years we will have logged about 1000 hours, the point where Goleman, Davidson, and other researchers begin to notice significant differences in brain responses. These differences become quite dramatic when they watch the brains of those who have 10,000 to 30,000 hours or more of meditation practice. These "Olympic" meditators can drop in and out of meditation within a minute, and can do so repeatedly. Even more interesting, they do not prepare themselves emotionally to feel pain, by anticipating it in the way the rest of us do (Goleman & Davidson, 2017).

Subjects in one of their experiments received a 10-second painful (but not tissue-damaging) burn after a 10-second heat warning. Highly advanced meditators' brains responded only to the painful stimulus itself and then let it go. A control group of newly taught meditators began responding to the 10-second heat warning as if it were pain, and they even maintained this "sense of pain" throughout the 10-second rest periods between tests (Goleman & Davidson, 2017).

MRIs of the advanced meditators' brains showed that the parts of their brains that sense pain sensed it more strongly than the control group, but the parts of their brain that "worried" about pain reacted very little. The advanced meditators showed similar responses to suffering. They became intensely present to the suffering of others (in photos) and let those emotions go almost immediately. These abilities to be fully present in the moment show up in measurable changes of brain function after a minimum of 10,000 hours of practice, and improve noticeably after 30,000 hours of practice (Goleman & Davidson, 2017).

Of course, meditation may not engage our interest in the way it does for people who find the time to spend an hour a day in meditation or attend weeks and even years of advanced training in such practices. What does catch our attention on a daily basis? Do we see improvements in our overall health as a result of practicing these skills? Have we logged 30,000 hours building any specific skill?

Certainly, most of us have put an hour a day over the course of decades in many tasks, mostly work-related. When we pursue such physical and mental skill building practices we can reach a generally very happy state, psychologist Mihaly Csikszentmihalyi called "flow." Neurologist, Allan Hamilton, discusses how this state evolves out of attention and practice. Success expert, Malcolm Gladwell, has written that in order to make a contribution to any field we must put in an average of 10,000 hours of practice. He calls this "the 10,000 hour rule" (Hamilton, 2018).

Parenting certainly gets better with practice. Ask any grandparent about what they learned through those wonderful moments when their child's face brightened with understanding and delight, as well as the times they drew a line in the sand, lost their temper, or used force and had to live with regret and guilt afterwards. Grandchildren often get the benefit of their grandparents' heightened attention and practice.

Home cooking gets better with practice, as do most job skills, those that require mental and physical skills as well as those we consider rote or meaningless. We may not love to spend 15 minutes a day decluttering, but if we persist for a month of this habit (7 hours) we will find it gets easier. We may not love cleaning the house, but the person who does it daily as a way to make a living will log enough hours to become an expert and will do a more efficient job than those of us who haven't come close to that magic 1000 to 10,000 hours of brain-changing skill.

I always ask children I evaluate, "What do you want to do when you grow up?" Usually, I get an answer right away, up until they reach the end of primary school and learn from well-meaning adults that their choice requires a level of expertise and training they may never hope to achieve. I believe this information can rob the world of these children's talents and interest.

My all-time favorite answer came from a child with special needs, a young woman who did not even know her age. (She was off by 2 years.) She was quite clear about what she wanted to do with her life: peacock farming. I imagine her today among a flock of brightly colored birds, scattering grain, cleaning pens, and cuddling fluffy peachicks. I can only hope her adoring parents, who had no idea where she got this desire, helped make her dream possible. The world could be a better place with peacock farmers in it.

I also ask adults struggling with depression over a lifetime of regrets, "What did you want to do in kindergarten?" So begins our quest to bring more joy and hope into their present life, one currently filled with "have to," "should," and endless, unfinished "to do" lists.

Finding time to spend an hour a day developing a skill we love could bring us the same remarkable results in brain function that meditation provides, and I believe it will take us on a similar journey. Fishermen (and women), knitters, gardeners, woodworkers who use hand tools, artists, and musicians all report feeling "flow" when doing repetitive, skill-building tasks.

We may not make our living performing these skills, but we can still make them part of our daily lives. In *Your Money or Your Life: Transforming Your Relationship with Money and Achieving Financial Independence,* Joe Dominguez and Vicki Robin recount the story of a nurse who felt constrained by the insufficient income he received doing the nursing work he loved. He took a better-paying job delivering fuel oil to rural customers. He offered to measure vital signs, organize medication, and communicate with health care providers for his ailing elderly clients as he made his delivery rounds. He found joy in his unpaid work, and provided for his own family at the same time.

Your Money or Your Life engaged the simplicity movement from its first publication in 1992 and has stayed in print. This movement, also known as "voluntary poverty," has had many manifestations over the centuries while people grappled with having too much stuff and feeling chained to those possessions by economic necessity.

Charles Eisenstein's *Sacred Economics: Money, Gift, and Society in the Age of Transition* also looks at where we have been in terms of money and work, and he uses these ideas to imagine "the more beautiful world our hearts know is possible" when we learn to separate what we do best from the money we need to make for basic survival.

Many of us feel grief when we listen to endless reports on the state of climate change; the extinction of beautiful species; and the loss of wild spaces, empty lots, community gardens, and small farms to housing developments and strip malls. We feel grief for people we have lost to death, drugs, disagreements, or relocation. We feel grief for our own missed opportunities. All of us grasp and hold on to things as a stand-in for good times, loved ones, and a sense of hope. The brain changes Goleman and Davidson found in advanced meditators made it seem effortless for them to let go of their attachments to pain and grief (Goleman & Davidson, 2017).

A number of creative writers have embraced the challenges of the greatly altered lifestyles we face through climate change, loss of fossil fuels, and collapse of the world we know. Like those who survived and thrived at the end of the Bronze Age, they can see something to move toward with equanimity once we let go of our attachments to stuff. In *World Made by Hand*, James Howard Kuntsler portrays a former stockbroker who makes furniture for his neighbors in exchange for baskets, meat, and dentistry performed with a bicycle-powered drill. John Michael Greer's *Retrotopia* takes us to a country in the Ohio Valley where 40 years of embargo by neighboring countries has resulted in a wholly different economy and reuse of older technologies such as canals, radio, horse-powered plows, and even microwaves to provide its inhabitants with a great deal of comfort, security, and beauty.

When we change our stories about work, we change our beliefs and begin healing centuries-old wounds from industrial-driven lifestyles and religious doctrines that emphasize suffering and separation. These practices generally serve a few at the expense of many. They depend on ignoring what our body, mind, and spirit are telling us to do to ease our own pain and grief, as well as that of our family, friends, and neighbors. We want to see our work create objects of beauty and function, help others, and leave behind a world where our children can thrive. Doing so integrates body, mind and spirit. It places us back on a path where work serves our health instead of making us sick.

Inspiration and Elimination: The Healing Power of Metal Energies

Our lungs and skin take in Metal elements through contact with air. Along with the colon they provide a protective barrier that sorts elements out, keeping what nourishes us and allowing us to eliminate those toxins we cannot avoid.

Our health depends on the quality of air we breathe and absorb through our skin. Breathing also activates our immune system. The lungs filter and eliminate toxins from the air. Some studies have found that teaching people meditation practices, many of which focus on breathing, enhances their immune responses (Goleman & Davidson, 2017).

Although we do everything we can to stop a runny nose, skin eruptions, and diarrhea, these symptoms mean our bodies are getting rid of toxins—material, emotional, and energetic. Our hair and sweat glands assist us with detoxification.

Hair analysis reveals what elements we have eaten and absorbed from the environment. Archaeologists use hair analysis to determine both food and environmental conditions surrounding the ancient people they study. Some people remove hair follicles and sweat glands for cosmetic reasons. Often women of childbearing age, striving to meet contemporary standards of beauty, undergo these painful procedures. Hair and sweat play an important role in detoxification, and these procedures can directly impact both fertility and health of mothers and babies.

Our noses have the ability to make almost instantaneous chemical analysis of the air we smell and breathe. One relatively short nerve picks up stray electrons or molecular shapes and carries that information directly to the limbic system for analysis and from there to parts of the cortex involved in actions (Burr, 2003). Since our memories and emotions reside in the limbic system, we often have visceral reactions to scents.

Most of us instantly recognize the smell of an elementary school and have either positive or negative responses based on our experiences from school

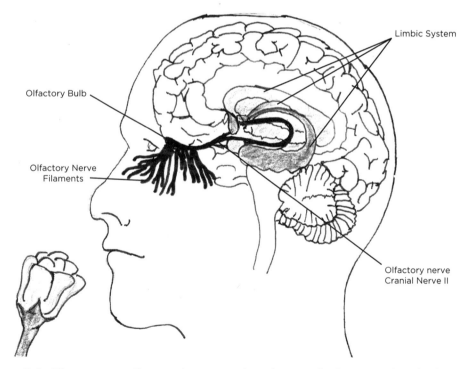

Figure 5.6   The nerve endings make a very short journey before entering the limbic system, where a complex arrangement of neural connections integrates this sense with memory, emotion, and our organs to help us choose everything from food to mates.

days. I have known people who judged the quality of a library by its scent—old paper and bindings have a very different scent from modern publications and electronic media. Aromatherapies can play a role in healing because of the complex connections in our olfactory sensory system.

Our large intestine, or colon, plays a big role in the final separation of nutrients, including water, from wastes. Many species of bacteria and other microorganisms live in the microbiome of our colon. These creatures help us break down hard-to-digest proteins like gluten and soy so that we can absorb important nutrients. Microscopic species that thrive on the copious amounts of sugar and flours in our diets have developed a reputation for causing or exacerbating inflammation underlying serious health conditions. Our colon plays a big role in our immune system, and we benefit from eating to keep a healthy microbiome. (See Chapter 3: Earth Energies.)

Crying, a common expression of grief, also reduces stress, makes us feel better, and appears to boost our immune system. A beautiful sunrise can bring us to tears, and those early morning hours when we dream also resonate with Metal energies. Giving ourselves permission to cry and opportunities to dream provides vital moments for inspiration.

In autumn we prepare to let go of the summer's warmth. We say goodbye to blooming and fruiting plants, as well as all but the hardiest leafy greens and edible roots. Herbalists often use plants that we associate with autumn to boost our immune systems and dry up excess mucus. Witch hazel, which blooms in late fall or winter, has long been used to tone and firm our skin, as a mild astringent. Also look for it as the main active ingredient in over-the-counter treatments for hemorrhoids. Spicy foods often make our noses run and our eyes tear, another way to access the healing properties of Metal energies through what we eat.

Eliminate Clutter: Preparing Space for Inspiration

Decluttering our lives from debris as well as emotions can have a visible effect on our surroundings as well as our health. As we make space for inspirational work, we can look for a decrease in upper respiratory symptoms such as colds and bouts of asthma. Take some "before" and "after" photos. Does our skin seem more radiant?

When our beliefs stay tethered to notions of illness caused by pathogens that only respond to medical interventions, we cut ourselves off from our own power to alter our health for the better. Could clearing our desks and cleaning out our closets make a difference in the number of colds we get? Run the experiment with yourself as the subject, N=1. Check your results.

Exercise 5.3: Try Making an Archaeological Expedition Into Our Lives

Unless we are one of the blessed Born Organized, we probably have piles—lots of them. We receive daily inundations of junk mail, packaging materials, important emails, bills, magazines, newspapers, and cool stuff someone bought on sale. It all has to go somewhere, and pretty soon we have quite the collection of stuff on every surface in our homes. Archaeologists love these kinds of collections, which they call middens. That's a polite, academic word for "trash heaps." When we begin our 5-to-15-minutes-a-day excavations into our own middens we find all sorts of lost treasures, just like archaeologists. We need to take those things we love out of our middens and put them where we can see them every day. We need to clear a space around them, like a savvy shopkeeper or museum curator. Then we can make our homes a showcase for what inspires us.

Aim for being able to walk into a room and take a deep breath of admiration at our own rich life full of beauty, useful tools, and reminders that inspire joy.

Exercise 5.4: Learn to Get Rid of Grief

Close to one-in-ten adults and one-in-eight adolescents feel depressed in the U.S. (National Institute of Mental Health, 2016). Depression saps our energy and makes it even harder to face the daily chores we do to keep body and soul together. That includes not having energy to take out the trash, sift through the junk mail, or wash dirty dishes in the sink.

While the idea of decluttering may seem liberating, the actual act of letting things go can put us on the couch for a major binge watch, complete with bowls of ice cream or chips to stuff down our feelings of grief. Treasures that lift our spirits sit right alongside stuff that puts us on a dark road, filled with memories of loss and regret. Pushing through that takes effort, willpower, and practice.

Many people recommend approaching depression by making a gratitude list, writing down everything good in our life on a daily basis. If this works for you, and it does for many, keep it up. When we display things that bring us joy, they serve as a physical gratitude list.

Gratitude doesn't work for everyone. Some of us have had some pretty awful stuff happen, and sometimes we keep reminders of those times in objects that should make us happy, but don't. Sometimes we need to express this grief and anger to make way for gratitude. Luckily for us, tossing stuff in the garbage can help with that, too.

Make a quick survey of your surroundings. What triggers grief, anger, or annoyance? Choose a particularly troublesome item and write the ugly thoughts it triggers on that object with a marker, or on a piece of paper attached to that object. Or, write the day's troubling thoughts on a piece of junk mail, then toss it in the garbage.

Find 5, 10, or 15 grief-triggering items, and get them out of the house. It rarely serves us to spend too long thinking about what to let go. Set a timer for 5, 10, or 15 minutes and grab whatever you can. Make a game of it. Do we get better with practice?

People who sit for hours in meditation without moving generally feel bodily pain at some point. They learn to focus on that pain until they can detach from it, and lots of people pay good money to spend a weekend, 10 days, or even years doing just this kind of daily practice. Freedom comes in befriending pain and observing it with detachment. (Goleman & Davidson, 2017).

Sometimes we need to focus on what we don't like in our surroundings and get rid of it. Sometimes we keep things we don't like, merely to save money. If we worry about these kinds of issues we might want to do a quick cost comparison with the kinds of illness produced by the stress of having too much, either clutter or regrets. I have a friend who always says, "This will cost much less than a heart bypass," to give himself permission to spend money on some activity that he knows will help him feel better immediately and improve his health in the long run. Getting rid of clutter can save us thousands of dollars in health care costs associated with allergies and the resulting inflammation they cause.

Laugh, cry, shout, and scream. Get rid of all that useless stuff.

Set an Intention and Do It: Build Willpower 15 Minutes a Day

When strong feelings come up during decluttering, we often just need to push through. As with meditation practice, the longer we do it the easier it gets. Structure helps. Set your intention with a timer. Research has shown positive effects from meditation in about 15 minutes, so keep breathing and keep going until your timer chimes at the end of 15 minutes. Stay focused.

Exercise 5.5: Set an Intention and Harness the Power of Metal Energy to Get the Job Done

We can use a mechanical timer with a chime or the timer app on our mobile phone with a special ringtone, whichever is easiest or gives us the most pleasure. Each day before beginning to de-clutter we need to spend a few minutes standing in front of our Healing Compass to remind ourselves of why we want to declutter our home. Do we want better health, more joy, or a clean place to entertain friends and family? Focus on breathing in that specific intention, and breathing out everything that gets in our way of achieving it. Take 5 deep breaths. Set the timer. Place it in the West where Metal energy is strongest.

Everyone who meditates loses focus at the beginning. Treat this practice as an action meditation. When we get sidetracked on an object filled with memories, we need to put that aside and move on to an easier target. Breathe in. Breathe out. Scan the room. Focus on a specific surface. Keep going until the chimer chimes.

We need to enjoy what we do, or the results that they bring, and hopefully both. Use strategies to make it fun. Weigh that bag of clutter before throwing it in the trash or taking it to a recycling center. Keep track of how much weight you eliminate each day on a calendar or Worksheet 5.5.

Make sure that clutter gets out of the house and out of the car if it's going to a recycling center. We want to eliminate the weight, not lose it. When we lose weight, there's always a chance we might find it again!

Worksheet 5.5: Keeping Track of Progress Eliminating Clutter Weight

Write the start date in a corner of one of the boxes on the first row. Continue the numbers sequentially in the boxes that follow until you have filled out 30 days of dates. Write down how many pounds of clutter get eliminated each day. Whenever you find a hidden treasure to display or use write it down in the box. Make some stars around it. Use the back of the sheet to keep a gratitude list of all you have found that brings you joy.

Sunday	Monday	Tuesday	Wednesday	Thursday	Friday	Saturday

We can give ourselves a reward for getting rid of stuff. Relax, put our feet up, drink a glass of water, and watch the wind blow or call a friend. Using a daily reward after a decluttering session can help us keep going. We must remember to give ourselves a pat on the back for every day we do this, as well as forgive ourselves for lapses. They happen to us all. It takes about thirty days to get a habit in place. Keep going.

Make It Your Own: Whistle While You Work

Decluttering becomes a skill with practice. Along the way, we find out how to make it work for us. Whenever I need decluttering and cleaning inspiration,

I turn to my favorite cleaning guru, Marla "FlyLady" Cilley, author of *Sink Reflections.* Her book is full of encouragement and laughter, as is her website. Her motto, "You can do anything for 15 minutes," became a foundation for this practice.

Decluttering gurus can tell us how they do it, and some of those suggestions will work for us. We all need to find our own best ways. Check out other decluttering programs and cleaning systems. If we find something we like, incorporate it into our practice. Just remember, small changes get big results. Add them in manageable amounts. Grow our decluttering practice.

What kind of music helps us keep going? A strong beat generally moves the action along nicely. Try some sing-along music. Singing will help dispel the anxiety that comes from letting go of what we no longer need or want but feel we need to keep.

Gifts from others rank high on the list of stuff we keep but don't really want. Collections of anything usually contain more than a few gifts that we never would have bought for ourselves. Regift them, or take them to an organization that will pass them on to a good home. Kiss them. Feel the love that motivated that gift, and let it go with the same love.

We enjoy the treasures we can see and use every day. How many precious items get put away for special occasions and then get forgotten and never used? Unpack those boxes and cupboards. We deserve to use beautiful things every day. If we worry about precious things getting damaged, we never get to enjoy them. Dishes break. Fine clothing becomes stained. Nice furniture gets shabby with daily use. The same thing happens to our bodies, but unlike these things our cells have the ability to repair and replace themselves.

Our bodies do age, like every other living thing. We see that in autumn as leaves fall and plants wither. With care our wounds heal most of the time. We get to decide if we want to spend our precious life avoiding every risk, or engaging our mind, body, and spirit in adventures that bring us joy and experience. We need to trust ourselves to make these choices, accept the consequences, and move on.

We have the ability to hold on to our memories of good times without hoarding every item that reminds us of those times. We have the ability to get better when we can let go of mistakes and regrets. Self-confidence comes with practice. Create a space where inspiration flourishes.

Share It: Clean up the Neighborhood

We all live someplace where trash collects. Even our oceans have large patches of collected debris from our leftover and neglected waste. Cleaning up these massive islands of (mostly) plastic boggles our minds and crushes our will. Walking around our neighborhoods with a bag and some gloves provides us with exercise and connects us with the conscious universe as an ally, or friend. If we're feeling playful and imaginative we might even talk to the trees, bushes, and plants where trash tends to collect.

Try this practice in front of your house or apartment. At first we may get some funny looks from neighbors, especially if we're talking to the trees, but this gives us an opportunity to build the skill of self-confidence, detaching from what others think of us. As our neighborhood gets cleaner and prettier we may find that others begin to respond differently. They may join us or put in a few flowers. We may find the plants calling out to us for companions in the forms of birds, butterflies, and other pollinators. Lots of garden companies offer wild-flower seed mixes specific to geographical regions. When we plant these we get lots of low-care flowers that attract even more beauty to our homes. Take the chance to inspire your community.

Exercise 5.6: Decluttering with Children

Teaching children to get rid of things they no longer use will provide them with a practice that can serve them for life. Most cultures do not recommend meditation practice for children before adolescence, but a monthly practice of sharing toys and clothes with other children can plant the seeds of compassion and loving kindness that could grow into an adult meditation practice.

Loving-kindness meditation involves wishing yourself and others well-being, happiness, and ease from suffering. It creates a positive mood. Research has shown positive changes in the brain after as short a time as 8 hours of loving-kindness meditation. It makes the difference in feeling immobilized by another's suffering because we feel it as if it was our own, to reaching out to that person as a parent would to a child (Goleman & Davidson, 2017). The longer we practice loving-kindness meditations, the more active the "happiness" circuits of our brains become.

Children, who love and enjoy their toys and clothes, can pass that enjoyment on to other children. They can learn to winnow out the toys and clothes they love from those for which they may not have as strong an attachment, by focusing on sharing enjoyment.

The key to helping a child develop this form of loving kindness rests in allowing them to choose, without comment or judgment from others, which of their toys and clothes they want to share. It may wrench our hearts to see them part with an expensive gift we have given them, or something they have barely used. We need to stand back and let them begin to navigate this important practice on their own.

Note that loving-kindness practice always begins with compassion for self. Loving a particular toy or piece of clothing past its prime or age-appropriateness imbues that object with a powerful energy. We will learn more about Love in the next chapter, but most of us can remember the story of the *Velveteen Rabbit*, who became real because of a boy's love. That story will still bring me to tears. If we place a "share" box or bag in a child's room, we encourage them to play with the concept of loving kindness on a daily basis. Give them a finite goal of 5 to 15 items each month and watch how they choose what to release each month. They can teach us a great deal about our own abilities to detach from things.

Exercise 5.7: Decluttering with Elders

Nothing will make us a believer in the benefits of getting rid of stuff like cleaning out the home of a parent who has passed on or moved to a smaller residence. Sifting through books, magazines, letters, clothing, china, and all manner of seemingly meaningless collections helps us begin to question our own day-to-day choices of what to keep and what to throw or give away.

Often elders begin their collection process early in life, and it has become a life-long habit. Sometimes the collecting stands in as a means to stave off sadness from the uncontrollable losses they face: diminished senses; forgetfulness; deaths of spouse, friends, pets, and family. Sometimes stuff piles up when they no longer have the strength or will to move it.

Regardless of the reason why they have so much stuff, it results in health problems. Cluttered environments contribute to upper respiratory ailments, falls, and depression, all of which affect elders even more seriously than younger people.

When attempting to help another person with decluttering, go slowly and have them decide when and what to let go. Each time you visit, offer to carry out trash, or take items to charity. This will offset their lack of strength and endurance for these tasks.

When we see something useful and unused, we might suggest who among family and friends could get immediate benefit from having that item. Knowing something we love will go to another person who treasures it may make it easier for an elder to let go. Getting used to that idea may take a bit of time. If possible, make sure elders get to see a photo of the item with its new owner in its new home. A concrete representation of sharing joy can go a long way toward alleviating elders' sadness and help them share more items in the future.

When collecting stuff constitutes a lifelong habit, let go of your own expectations or desires for change in an elder's lifestyle. Such radical deviations in behavior rarely occur late in life. Many elders clearly recognize that their stuff puts them at risk for falls. They may even see that their stuff makes it harder to breathe, walk, and have friends and family come to visit. In these cases we must make loving kindness part of our own practice, and let go of our attachment to changing their behavior.

CHAPTER 6

Fire Energies

Make Friends! Passion and Process in Relationship

God sent Noah the rainbow sign. No more water.
There'll be fire next time.

—JAMES BALDWIN

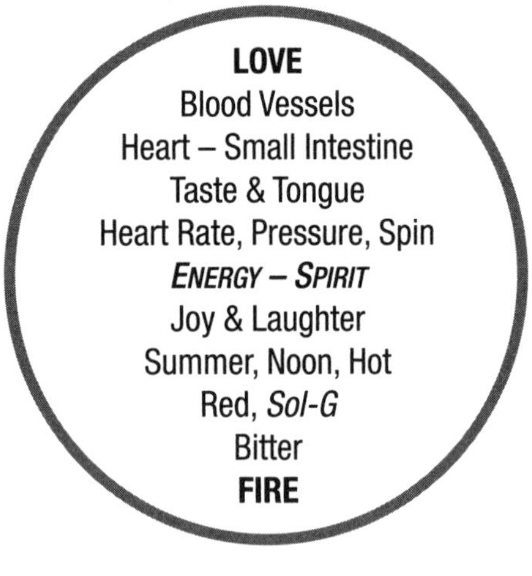

FIRE BURNS. IT heats our food, warms our hearths, lights our darkness, and always fascinates us. Without sunshine we would have no life at all. We make a complete circuit around our own yellow star every year. The sun, constant maker of our days, often goes unnoticed until a heat wave shrivels crops and costs us our lives. We complain when the sun hides behind clouds, even when those clouds bring much needed, nourishing rain. Total eclipses give birth to stories, myths, legends, scientific study, and silly nonsense.

LOVE
Blood Vessels
Heart – Small Intestine
Taste & Tongue
Heart Rate, Pressure, Spin
ENERGY – SPIRIT
Joy & Laughter
Summer, Noon, Hot
Red, *Sol-G*
Bitter
FIRE

Figure 6.1 Life Aspects Associated with Fire Energies

Death-defying phoenixes rise from their own ashes. Devils live in a fiery underground hell. Dragons breathe fire. Lions, horses, salamanders, and fireflies have Fire energy. Prometheus gave humans the gift of fire, according to the ancient Greeks, and paid the price by being chained to a rock on Mount Caucasus, where an eagle came every day to consume his heart or liver until Hercules finally rescued him. Vestal virgins kept an eternal flame burning in ancient Roman temples. Anyone who has ever attempted to start a fire by rubbing two sticks together or even striking flint rocks can attest to the usefulness of a constant source of fire for cooking, heating, and light.

From before we became *Homo sapiens*, some 200,000 years ago, we began gathering around a fire to share warmth, food, and companionship (Gowlett, 2016). Cooperation around a fire defined our beginnings. It may also define our dying out, or evolution to another species, as we stand on the brink of our own destruction with the burning of fossil fuels and splitting of atoms.

Like the mythic phoenixes who rise from the ashes of their own nests, we may find ourselves in another era, transformed, in the way dinosaurs became birds over the course of hundreds of millions of years. Like humans, many birds live cooperatively in groups called flocks; or murders, if they happen to be crows; and exaltations, if they happen to be larks.

With us or without us, the Earth will continue its revolutions around the sun for trillions of years after we are gone. Despite slogans urging us to "save the planet," it is really our own lives we must save. And, more likely than not, we will do so in the time-honored means of gathering around a fire—some external source of heat and light—where we can share food, ideas, companionship, and care for each other

Exercise 6.1: Making a Conscious Connection with Fire Energy

For this exercise we must light a candle or make a small fire in a fireplace or other fire-safe container such as an incense burner.

Place the small flame in the South on the Healing Compass. As we watch the flames . . .What do we notice?

Flames can often mesmerize. They are sometimes so entrancing we forget to stay aware, to make sure that Fire stays in the home we have provided.

Try feeding Fire some small scraps of paper, wood, green leaves, metal. What happens? Be ready with water or a wet towel to cover the flames should they escape from their safe container. What can Fire teach us?

Search for "Fire stories" both myths and true stories. Think of songs with fire references? "Come on baby, light my fire!"

How can we use our imagination to tell us about Fire energy?

Practice Passion: The Process of Community Building

This habit will reconnect us with our tribe, those one hundred and fifty or so people whose lives intertwine with ours. In *150 Strong: A Pathway to a Different Future*, Rob O'Grady points out that in order to achieve sustainability we must reconcile our individual differences in collective communities with common goals. He proposes that the best way we can do this is to connect with our own 150 people and consciously maintain those connections.

We all have people in our lives. We have family, friends, coworkers, and people we encounter regularly in a variety of social and service networks. We get steady bursts of our happy hormone, oxytocin, when we engage with others in these networks. A whole host of health benefits arise from these connections. Our practice for this chapter focuses on how to maintain, rekindle, and develop those relationships.

We will do this by identifying and making an effort to physically connect with people from our "tribe," our network of 150. We will aim to share food or beverages with another person three times a week, to meet for playful interactions with a group once a week, and to call a distant friend or family member once a week. In this way we strengthen our networks and build social capital, our strongest link to health and happiness.

Happy Talk: Our Brains on Dopamine and Oxytocin

Many millions of years of evolution have gone into making it possible for beings, plants and animals, to live in cooperative communities for their collective benefit. In vertebrates, the brain and nervous system plays a particularly important role. Scientists have only scratched the surface of how this works, but we do know that language, oxytocin, endorphin, dopamine, and blood flow play significant roles.

So far, scientists have found that the ability to imitate vocal sounds occurs in only in a few mammals and birds. This ability seems to have evolved independently in humans, bats, whales, dolphins, sea lions, elephants, songbirds, parrots, and hummingbirds. The ability has direct links to our happy hormones, oxytocin and dopamine. These two hormones keep us connected and goal-directed.

Imitation makes use of some specialized neurons in our brains called mirror neurons. Scientists find that when primates (people, monkeys, and apes) observe other primates do a goal-directed task, the same neurons light up in the observers as in those doing the task. One reason we may find it enjoyable to watch sports or drama is to see other people getting hits of dopamine, serotonin, and oxytocin. As their neurons light up for making the basket, leading a team to victory, or getting the love of their life, those of us watching get a similar hormonal rush (Breuning, 2017).

Mirror neurons mean that we have special abilities that predispose us to copy behaviors. These types of neurons form an important foundation for learning. Mirror neurons fire in response to auditory and visual stimuli, as well as movements and emotions. The ability to move from copying these sounds to improvising and using them for communication happens in only a few species of birds and mammals (Levy, 2012). Scientists also find that doing this stimulates both dopamine (achieving a goal) and oxytocin (connecting with another being) (Theofanopoulou, Boeckx, & Jarvis, 2017).

Our ability to successfully reproduce sounds, as babies do when they babble, and later reform those sounds into language involves many complex neural pathways through our neocortex, limbic system, and nerves to muscles involved in making sound. It generally takes humans 2 to 3 years to achieve this. It doesn't happen in babies and young children separated from other human contact. Also, for reasons we still don't entirely understand, it doesn't happen, or stops happening, in children diagnosed with many autism spectrum disorders.

Bird brains look very different from human brains, but when scientists look at those birds who can sing songs with variety, like songbirds, parrots, and hummingbirds, they find that their brains make similar circuits that trigger both dopamine and oxytocin. All of these circuits depend on important connections in the birds' forebrain, which has similar characteristics with our neocortex, the part of our brain that accomplishes complex tool use and language (Theofanopoulou, Boeckx, & Jarvis, 2017).

Birds evolved quite differently from mammals, though both of us come from the time of dinosaurs. Birds have a much closer relationship to dinosaurs, and since we know that birds take care of their young, many paleontologists hypothesize that at least some species of dinosaurs took care of their young as well. Mammals were already becoming different from birds back in the day, some 300 million years ago, when our ancestors shared a living space with seedless plants we now burn as coal. As millions of years went by we became even more different than birds. Bird's brains are much smaller than ours, but in songbirds the part of their brain that corresponds with our neocortex has a very high density of neurons. This leads scientists to hypothesize that they use language to communicate and connect with others of their kind (Olkowicz et al., 2016).

Birds and mammals have descended from ancestors who survived two mass extinctions, the Triassic-Jurassic and the Cretaceous-Paleogene. The Triassic-Jurassic has been blamed on an asteroid impact some 200 million years ago. Before that extinction event, mammal species outnumbered dinosaur species. For about 130 million years after that, dinosaurs proliferated and achieved their legendary size. The Cretaceous-Paleogene extinction, blamed on a combination of volcanic activity, asteroid impact, and climate change, happened about 65 million years ago. After that, dinosaurs disappeared completely, leaving behind reptiles and birds to carry on. Each one of these extinctions took millions and millions of years to reach completion. By comparison, a human life of 100 years could produce four generations: children by 25 years, grandchildren by 50; great-grandchildren by 75; and great-great grandchildren by 100. A million years would produce 250,000 generations, enough time for humans to become significantly different from the ancestors we share with Neanderthals, but certainly outside the scope of memory, except where that gets encoded in DNA as instinct. In fact, even Stonehenge, which took roughly 1000 years and 4,000 generations to complete, has dimmed beyond retrieval in our collective memory some 20,000 generations later.

> *Beliefs create thoughts.*
> *Thoughts create emotions.*
> *Emotions create actions.*
> *Actions create health.*

If we *believe* survival of the fittest means the strongest individual needs to take what they want and fight off any competitors to win the game of evolution, we may *think* that our lives matter more than anyone else, certainly more than any other species sharing our planet. We must grab whatever we want and need to *enjoy* now. No need to waste time helping others or thinking about children and grandchildren. Leave that to the weaker, less forceful among us.

If we *believe* survival depends on each species' ability to cooperate and support the environments that give them life, we may *imagine* ourselves living in a vibrant and sentient web of continuous creation, destruction, and creation. Learning about those who share our planet and contribute to the air we breathe, the water we drink, and the food we eat connects us to a constant source of life and regular moments of *joy*. We build sustainable communities where we can raise our children and grandchildren to pass on both our genetic and learned wisdom.

Certainly, we need to take climate change and impending extinctions seriously, but we also need to understand that our personal emotional drama and trauma happens on a much smaller time scale, one we can manage, especially if we have a community to support us through political upheavals and natural disasters. Spending time together, building bonds through compassionate action, touch, and language, gives us a focus for today. It brightens our days and nights with joy. It also enhances our personal and species survival.

We depend on the help of friends, family, and neighbors to get through all manner of natural disasters and personal troubles. The bonds we build in community will ensure getting through impending changes in climate that threaten the loss of natural resources, such as breathable air, drinkable water, and access to food. Preserving the ecosystems that give us life, ensures the continuation of the next generation, and the ones that come after.

Exercise 6.2: Changing a Belief

Take a moment to imagine the future, your own, or even further into the potential worlds of our children and grandchildren. Do these thoughts elicit excitement for untold possibilities or fears of loss? If our thoughts elicit fear we need to spend some time examining the beliefs underlying those thoughts and exercise our creativity to imagine a happier scenario.

After all we are making up our own future story. It hasn't happened yet and we can control an imaginary ending. We can't cheat by ignoring our fears. Fear alerts us to danger and we need to listen to it. We must confront our fears and examine them from every angle like a puzzle until we see a way through to that happy ending.

We can light a small candle or fire in the South of the Healing Compass, as directed in Exercise 6.1. We can spend as long as we like pondering the puzzle of finding a happy ending. It may take one session or many. When we find a happy ending, that positive focus can change our life all the way down to our DNA.

Thinking with the Heart-Mind

In 1992, Richard Davidson, one of the authors of *Altered Traits*, and a team of scientists carried several hundred pounds of brain-measuring equipment (EEG electrodes and amplifiers, computer monitors, video recording equipment, batteries, and generators) on a three-day hike up narrow Himalayan mountain paths to the Dalai Lama's residence in exile. Once there, they set up their equipment in hopes of measuring what happens in the brains of long-time meditators. Sadly for them, after such an arduous trip, all of the monks refused to volunteer for measurement. In a last-ditch attempt to show the monks how the equipment worked, the scientists gave a live demonstration on one of their colleagues.

Two hundred monks attended this demonstration endorsed by the Dalai Lama. When the team presented their colleague with all the electrodes attached to his head the assembly of monks burst into loud laughter. At the time Davidson believed that the monk's laughter related to the funny looking wires, but he later found out that the placement of wires on the man's head had caused all the hilarity.

The scientists had told the monks they wanted to measure what happened during *lojong*, a form of meditation focused on developing compassion. The monks associated this form of meditation with the heart, not the head, and the absurdity of trying to measure what happens in the heart with wires attached to the head caused a universal sense of laughable absurdity. Some 15 years later, Davidson found measurable connections between this form of meditation and heart function (Goleman & Davidson, 2017).

A loving-kindness meditation, like *lojong*, begins with focusing on the meditators' own feelings of distress. As these calm with breathing and visualizations of various kinds, the meditator's focus shifts outward in ever-widening circles. We imagine sharing what brought us relief from suffering for the people we know and love. Then we share with our neighbors, fellow citizens, and even our enemies, eventually including all sentient life on the planet.

People who learn a form of loving-kindness meditation can increase good feelings and a sense of social connection in as little as 7 minutes. After twenty 10-minute sessions of a web-based loving-kindness meditation program, participants feel more relaxed and give more to charity than people who spend the same amount of time doing light exercise and stretching. After 8 hours, transitory brain changes begin to show up in measurements. After 16 hours, people can shift away from usually inflexible biases toward those different than themselves (Goleman & Davidson, 2017).

The results of practicing loving-kindness and compassion meditation don't just help develop empathy, they also show a tendency to produce more telomerase, an enzyme that protects chromosomes and slows down aging. A pilot study of women with 4 years of regular practice in loving-kindness meditation showed that they had longer telomeres (the part that holds chromosomes together and keeps them from unraveling) (Hoge et al., 2013).

We have other indications of the positive health effects gained from social engagement as well. One of these, an interesting long-term study performed at Montefiore Hospital in the Bronx, New York, looked at a cohort of 469 people aged 75 and older who were in good health with no signs of dementia. The researchers followed this group for about twenty-one years. During that time, 124 people developed dementia of various types, mostly Alzheimer's (61 people) and vascular dementia (30 people). The *New England Journal of Medicine* published their study, "Leisure Activities and Dementia in the Elderly" in 2003. A popular meme that identifies dancing as a preventative for dementia comes from this study.

The study identified leisure activities as either cognitive or physical in nature. Most studies of this kind do seem to focus on those two categories, because the media frequently trumpets the importance of both physical exercise and mental stimulation as powerful antiaging strategies. I propose looking at this excellent study's results from another perspective, social activities, which makes its way into research far less often. Those studies I have found usually define social activities as those which involve simply interacting with other people. As we take a look at some of the results of this study I want to showcase those activities that involve not just interaction, but the kinds of "low stakes," playful interactions defined in Chapter 2 of this book, which discussed the importance of having fun to relieve stress and inflammation.

Enjoyment of a leisure activity makes the frequency of doing it much more likely, whereas doing something that's "good for us" may ensure some initial involvement that deteriorates over time. Ask anyone who has ever signed up for a gym membership in January. When we look at Table 6.1 we can see the three activities with a hazard ratio that falls below 0.5 (which means half as likely to get dementia compared to the rest of the people they studied). These are dancing, playing board games, and playing a musical instrument. These seem like fun activities to me. It's unlikely that anyone over 75 years of age would have someone nagging them to practice playing music, something that takes much of the fun out of it for young people. All three of these activities generally involve social interaction as well.

Table 6.1: Which Leisure Activities Work Best to Keep Us from Developing Dementia.

Activities that seem to protect against developing dementia (from best to least protective)	Participated once a week or less			Participated several times a week				
	# Who got dementia	Total who did this	Hazard ratio	# Who got dementia	Total who did this	Hazard ratio	Low	High
Dancing	99	339	1.00	25	130	**0.24**	0.06	0.99
Board games	108	366	1.00	16	103	**0.26**	0.17	0.57
Playing a musical instrument	120	452	1.00	4	17	**0.31**	0.11	0.90
Crossword puzzles	117	407	1.00	7	62	**0.59**	0.34	1.01
Reading	40	87	1.00	84	382	**0.65**	0.43	0.97
Walking	19	65	1.00	105	404	**0.67**	0.45	1.05
Swimming	108	386	1.00	16	83	**0.71**	0.22	2.29
Babysitting	114	429	1.00	10	40	**0.81**	0.11	6.01
Housework	39	106	1.00	85	363	**0.88**	0.60	1.20
Writing	104	382	1.00	20	87	**1.00**	0.61	1.67
Team games	120	450	1.00	4	19	**1.00**	0.22	2.29
Group discussions	117	437	1.00	7	32	**1.06**	0.61	1.67
Group exercise	88	330	1.00	36	139	**1.18**	0.72	1.94
Climbing stairs	44	153	1.00	80	316	**1.55**	0.96	2.38
Bicycling	116	443	1.00	8	26	**2.09**	0.97	4.49

Source: Based on J. Verghese et al., Leisure activities and dementia in the elderly, *N Engl J Med.* 2003 Jun 19; 348(25):2508–16.

We usually read and do crossword puzzles alone. We can go walking or swimming alone or with someone else. These four activities still sound like fun to me, and they seem to reduce the chance of developing dementia, though not as much as the top three.

Babysitting and housework still come in below 1.00 in the hazard ratio, so they presumably have some minimally protective effect. Of course some people actually enjoy housework, and babysitting for children we like has the potential for fun.

Writing, team games like bowling, and group discussions don't seem to make much difference with a hazard ratio of 1.00. These all require some work. Group discussions among white, middle-class New Yorkers (who made up the majority of those in this research study) could be fun or stressful. Imagine preparing to discuss a book in a club where participants like to one-up each other with their academic expertise and scintillating insight. Instead of those fun dopamine and oxytocin bursts, we'd be competing to see who could get the most serotonin bursts of recognition for brilliance. I've sat in those book clubs, and I can tell you they aren't my idea of fun.

Then we get to group exercise, climbing stairs, and bicycling. These three activities actually seem to increase our risk for developing dementia—and yet health care professionals often encourage us to do these far more often than the first three.

Our Healing Compass could help us predict that those activities we enjoy would be good for our heart. When we participate in activities out of fear, it can deplete rather than build our energy, in the same way that lack of sleep does, since the emotion of fear, like sleep, resonates with Water energy. Overthinking and anxiety also slow down our digestive system and push us toward those sweets that have links to both diabetes and Alzheimer's. Engaging in joyful activities, resonates positively with our heart, and our longevity might increase, something the research on telomerase would support.

Of course, we all have different activities that we enjoy, but when I look at studies like this one I'm reminded that having fun with friends and family has very positive health gains.

Passion and Process: The Healing Power of Fire Energies

Our hearts bring us passion, and our guts let us process all that we take in. Oxytocin, the happy hormone we produce only in community, both soothes our heart and brings us joy. When we eat food, our guts, the 20 feet of our small intestine, process it, absorbing what nourishes us and passing on to the colon what needs to go. When we talk about having "guts" we usually mean "courage" a word with *coeur*, the French word for heart, at its root. Do we have the guts to take in joy?

Can we taste joy? Our tongues provide us with both the means to talk and the ability to chemically analyze our food by flavor. We have strong feelings about anything that goes into our mouths. Babies taste their world, first exploring it with lips and tongue. They learn to discriminate what feels good from all the rest. Each element has its own special flavor. Five Element Theory associates joy with bitter flavors: stimulating compounds like coffee, tea, and chocolate; leaves of radicchio, arugula, dandelion; flowers like saffron and rose petals; fruits of bitter melon and citrus; roots of turmeric and Jerusalem artichokes, also known as sun chokes. These foods cleanse the blood and stimulate the immune system.

If we *believe* that our heart is simply a pump, and our guts a necessary means toward digestion, we rarely *think* of them unless they give us pain. We *hate* them when they give us trouble, and we tend to *ignore* them until such time as we must drug them, cut into them, or even replace them with parts made in labs or from other bodies.

If we *believe* that our hearts connect us to the sun and our guts to the spirit of Fire, we *think* of them as precious, life-giving sources of love and caring. We *love* the way they keep the spark of life alive in us, and we *honor* them with compassion for ourselves and others.

Can we taste the warmth of the sun or a summer's day? Feel the sun's rays while relaxing in a hammock with a friend or lover? Have we laughed and screamed with a friend on the Ferris wheel or tilt-a-whirl at an amusement park? Our hearts and guts want to live in that world where we laugh and take pleasure in doing absolutely nothing useful. We need to take them to places and moments of joy as often as we can. Put your left hand over your heart and your right hand over your guts. Give thanks to the light in your heart and the fire in your belly. Keep their flames burning brightly. Pay attention when they speak to you in symptoms. Take care of them with love.

Make Friends! Cultivating Our Tribe

Even though we can communicate instantaneously around the globe, we sometimes overlook the special warmth of face-to-face and hand-to-hand contact. This chapter's practice will help us regain and strengthen our ties to other people.

In *The Globalization of Addiction,* Bruce Alexander puts forth a powerful argument that psychosocial integration, our sense of community, provides us with the strongest antidote to addiction. Spending enjoyable time with friends and family helps us build communities that inoculate us against the need to use addictive behaviors or substances, whether it's shopping, internet poker, or drugs (Alexander, 2011). We face an epidemic of opioid abuse in the United States, and many other countries have similar problems. Sugar and fast food addictions have created epidemic levels of obesity and diabetes, and these problems affect most countries around the world. Human trafficking has become an important concern for the United Nations, and as I write this we see the related issue of sexual harassment wreaking havoc in the worlds of media and politics.

This is not the world our hearts want to see. We want to feel secure in our homes, walking our streets, caring for our loved ones, and leaving behind a world of beauty and harmony for our children. The obstacles to doing these things often seem insurmountable, but we can begin to solve them in our own circles of engagement, one cup of tea, one meal, one card game, and one phone call at a time.

Exercise 6.3: Try Finding Your Tribe of 150

Get a big piece of paper and a pencil, or use Worksheet 6.3. Write your name in the center circle or the center of a blank page and make a small circle around it.

The next circle will contain our family members. Write in the names of immediate family and in-laws, if any. We may have family members with whom we no longer associate, and for good reasons, but write their names in anyway. Put brackets around the names of those with whom we do not have any current contact. They take up emotional space, even if we never speak to them.

Make a third circle around the first two and put the names of good friends, the people who "have our back," the ones we can go to for money, help, or comfort when the world starts falling apart around us.

Make a fourth circle and write the names of people we see or communicate with almost every day—neighbors, colleagues, people who touch our lives on a daily basis.

Make a fifth circle and write the names of people we communicate with on some kind of superficial level. Usually our social media friends outnumber 150. We can go to those lists of friends and copy names—or better yet, write the names that matter from memory.

A sixth circle could include people we see regularly at stores or places of worship, or those who provide regular services like delivering mail and picking up trash. We might not know their names yet, but we can learn them.

Count the names. Stop at 150, or whenever you can no longer think of anyone else to include. Take a look at the tribe you have assembled.

Take a look at the inner circles of names. When did we last sit down over a beverage or a meal with any of these people? Some of us have the good fortune to sit down to family meals every day. If we're not that lucky, then this practice will open our hearts to the benefits of breaking bread or sharing a beverage with others.

We can start by making contact with some of the people from the inner circles whom we haven't contacted in a while. A phone call to those far away can rekindle relationships. We can invite people who live nearby to share a meal or beverage with us. Some coffeehouses and restaurants have tables for chess or checkers. Invite a friend to join in a game. A pack of cards can fit in a pocket or purse. Can't remember how to play any card games? Bicycle Cards has an app for that (http://www.bicyclecards.com/rules/) Try it out. Have some laughs with a friend or two or three.

Worksheet 6.3: Finding our Tribe of 150

Write in the names of the people in our life, starting with ourself. Put brackets around any estranged family members. Our shared DNA connects us even if we have good reason to no longer communicate with them. Friends always have our back. We can count on neighbors and colleagues in an emergency. Acquaintances provide occasional but consistent touchpoints. We share our time and space with service workers and will benefit from learning their names and faces, in case of an emergency.

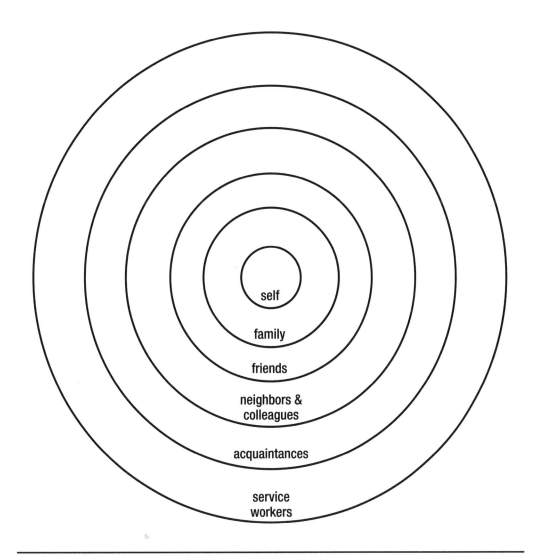

Exercise 6.4: Learn To Take Names and Play Games

Most of us see people on a daily basis and don't even acknowledge them. When we make our circles we can begin identifying people we might want to know by name. Will we invite them to dinner? Maybe not, but a quick, "Hello," or, "Good Morning," followed by their name won't hurt anyone. Sharing a smile and a wave will give us a burst of oxytocin that probably benefits our hearts more than coffee.

Why would we want to know these folks by name? Almost everyone who has ever experienced a blackout, storm, or other natural disaster has benefited from the kindness of strangers. Make a connection before it becomes imperative. In the meantime, enjoy those bursts of oxytocin from familiar passersby.

Part of this practice involves spending some time once a week playing with friends. Playing means interacting. Think of board games, cards, hiking, bowling, knitting, or sharing any activity we enjoy with others who enjoy it, too. We may have to research or buy some board games. We will have to call our friends and see who's up for a couple of hours of poker or a walk around the park. Setting up game nights takes work at first, but once established they take on a life of their own.

Exercise 6.5: Set an Intention and Do It: Have Courage for Relationships

If we're the type of people who keep to ourselves, it may feel strange or awkward to invite someone out to eat or to have a drink. Start small. We can offer to get someone a cup of coffee when we head out to get some for ourselves, then linger a moment and start a conversation. The weather, sports teams, shared work projects, and pets usually keep emotions fairly neutral or positive. Politics, religion, and sex generally lead to trouble in terms of conversation, especially at work. Jokes can lead to a laugh, or not, but they sure break the ice. Keep jokes "clean" – without references to sex, religion, or politics – until we know where others stand on these topics.

Pick neutral, safe, locations when asking someone we don't know well to share a meal or beverage. Neutral and familiar settings, like a nearby coffeshop or restaurant, tend to put people at ease. Even 15 minutes over coffee can open up other possibilities. We can ask questions and listen to other people's answers rather than spending the entire time talking about ourselves.

Make phone calls to far away friends and family. Texting and social media have their place for conveying quick information, but a longer call can warm the heart in a different way. Choosing times to call may present a challenge when people live in different time zones, but almost all of us love to hear from someone, even if we can't talk long at the moment. We establish connection and maintain relationships even with monthly or yearly calls to catch up. Make time to keep your tribe vital by putting in some energy.

Sharing meals or beverages, enjoying a shared game or activity with friends, and calling distant friends or relatives may feel awkward at first until we get comfortable with it. Pay attention to how it feels each time. Does it get easier?

We may need to give our self some time to set an intention before arranging these encounters. Use a version of Exercise 6.2: Changing A Belief to imagine a positive encounter and a happy ending. As we blow out our candle we let that vision go and have faith that our encounter will work out, even if not according to our pre-conceived plan.

Aim to share meals or beverages three times a week. Spend time enjoying an activity with friends, and call a distant friend or relative once a week. Do you see any changes in mood or health? Remember, we're conducting an experiment with a subject of one (N=1). Change it up in whatever way feels right to you. Focus on enjoying this practice. Remember joy and laughter keep the heart healthy. Keep track of progress by jotting brief notes on a calendar or Worksheet 6.5.

Worksheet 6.5: Keeping Track of Progress Making and Nourishing Friendships

Write the start date in a corner of one of the boxes on the first row. Continue the numbers sequentially in the boxes that follow until you have filled out 30 days of dates. Write down the first name of the person we shared any beverages, meals, or enjoyable time. B=beverage. M=meal or snack. G=game. C=conversation. If we had a good time we can draw in a few stars or hearts. Use the back of the sheet to write down any special details that don't fit in the box.

Sunday	Monday	Tuesday	Wednesday	Thursday	Friday	Saturday

Make It Your Own: Develop a Group of Regulars

When we make these practices part of our regular habits, magic happens. We start getting calls from others. People invite us out. We can become a regular event in other people's lives.

Game nights, hikes, or group meals, à la "girls' or boys' night out," take a few months to get going. When I lived in Tucson, Arizona, we had a 10-year, standing Friday girls' night out that encompassed a changing cast of characters and frequently included a male relative or friend of one of the regulars. We tried out new restaurants together and returned to old favorites. It more or less ran itself after the first year, as people would call to ask where we would meet. "GNO," as we called it, became a touch point for a wonderful community of friends. Many of the participants still meet regularly for game nights. I now live in New York City, and can rarely join them, but I love to hear that they still meet for games and meals.

After a month of practice, habits evolve. We find friendly meeting spots and the people who wait on us learn our names as we learn theirs. It warms the heart and impresses new people when we can walk into a place and get what we want without even ordering. We have seen it on TV and in movies, and we can make it happen in our own life.

The outer circles of our tribe of 150 start out kind of nebulous, with people we barely know, whose names we often forget. Then somewhere along the line we know their names and they know ours. We may not see them anywhere else, but we have touch points, places we could go if we needed the closeness of other people. The world seems friendlier. We feel more comfortable in our own body and our own neighborhoods. Nothing could give us any better heart's ease.

Share It: Widening the Circles

This practice revolves around sharing the warmth of community. Begin by sharing food and beverages. Pay some mind to keeping any regular group from becoming stuck in rigid patterns. We want to feel comfortable inviting new people from time to time, expanding our list of eating places, changing the scenery when hiking. Variety encourages us to keep our circles porous, flexible, and vital.

Rigid circles of friends that don't welcome potential new members run the risk of becoming gossipy and judgmental. Like hardening arteries, insular, unwelcoming groups can cause inflammation and even angry blowups.

Share your warmth with others, and watch the group grow. Members will come and go and return. With a flexible, self-sustaining group, even the person who originally called everyone together can take a night off without disappointing anyone.

Mix up venues from time to time as well. Businesses close. Wild places become shopping malls. We can mourn losses, but as with our bodies, we need to develop both flexibility and redundancy.

Share the love.

Exercise 6.6: Making Friends with Children

Children love to play games, from infancy onward. Within a few months after birth most infants have sufficiently integrated their senses of balance, touch, taste, smell, hearing, and vision so that they can take in the environment and begin focusing on the people who take care of them. We can start with lullabies and games like peek-a-boo and pat-a-cake. These activities help them develop both their vagal brake and language, two cornerstones for later social skills.

Toddlers have more play skills and can: toss around a ball or beanbag; play pretend with stuffed toys, dolls, or cars; read stories; sing songs; roughhouse gently; and play chase. Preschoolers can learn how to take turns and begin preferring to play with older children rather than adults. Two 4-year-olds can't play catch, but a 4-year-old and an 8-year-old do a splendid job. Eight-year-olds can toss a ball expertly enough for a younger child to catch, and they complain far less than adults when they have to run, jump, roll, and scramble for the wild tosses that a preschooler makes (Gray, 2013).

By the time kids start school they can learn to make rules, break rules, and "go along to get along" without any adult support or even supervision. These social skills developed on playgrounds and open areas will make it possible for them to navigate most home, school, and workplace encounters. As adults we need to provide these kinds of opportunities so our children can grow socially as well as intellectually and physically.

Having a weekly family game night with some neighbors or friends provides a wonderful opportunity to laugh and share good times, a place to model all those skills of getting along, and to hear the latest gossip from our children's circle of friends.

Family mealtimes also play an important part in keeping the home fires burning warm and bright. Multiple studies have shown that family meals improve grades and decrease teen drug use as well as teen pregnancies. This happens across all races and economic groups (Satter, 2008). Like game nights, family meals also provide the opportunity to hear who's bullying who, who's making trouble, and who helps other kids when they need it. This provides parents with important information they can use to help keep their children safe.

Exercise 6.7: Making Friends with Elders

Involving elder friends and relatives in game nights or mealtimes provides all of us with a host of important benefits. Elders keep their minds sharp and their hearts warm. Caretakers get to hear about health complaints before they get serious and learn about family history that provides both information and entertainment.

Enjoying time together keeps oxytocin flowing, something that elders might lack if they live alone and don't have the chance to share a conversation or a friendly hug with another person on a daily basis.

Dancing and board games appear equally protective against developing dementia, and that helps us all. Even elders who have slid into dementia can often do activities by habit that they have enjoyed for decades. Simple games, like solitaire, rummy, checkers, and Chutes and Ladders all require little short-term memory or strategy. They work for younger children and elders alike. Playing a familiar instrument after a lifetime of practice has so many sensory and movement connections that bypass the parts of the brain involved in short-term memory that elders can continue playing those pieces they know by heart even when they can't remember to get the mail or where they left their keys.

Daily or weekly phone calls provide an opportunity to check how an elder friend or relative is doing. Most elders appreciate short friendly calls that don't involve a constant barrage of questions requiring them to remember details they may have forgotten. Statements that invite comment or reminiscing always work best.

Sharing meals means we know that elders we care about get much-needed nutrition. Eating alone often means snacking rather than preparing a warm meal. Sending elders home with leftovers makes it possible for them to have one or more additional meals on their own. They can enjoy the company of others, even if they can't always hear or even understand what's being said. Keep them in conversations by asking questions that need a simple yes or no response. Avoid putting them on the spot to retrieve a lot of words they can't recall. Often we can get them to tell stories from their childhood or youth. We may have heard these stories before. Try to think about what makes the story so important that they repeat it. Ask some questions. Or have elders hang out with young children who can't listen to the same story enough times!

CHAPTER 7

Love Yourself!

Connect to Body's Wisdom

The body never lies.
—Nan Lu

Tuning in to our bodies gives us access to information about our health and the emotions driving our responses to the world around us.

Many people from diverse backgrounds agree that our bodies form the foundation for a conversation with the larger universe. Those who study *qigong* with Nan Lu hear him say this often. While searching for the origins of this quote, I found multiple sources. It led me to two books with similar titles, Mishio Kushi's, *Your Body Never Lies: The Complete Book of Oriental Diagnosis,* and Alice Miller's insightful, *The Body Never Lies: The Lingering Effects of Hurtful Parenting*. The quote has also been ascribed to Martha Graham and other dancers.

The body forms a direct link between us and the conscious universe. Tuning in to our bodies forms the foundation of Sustainable Health. Tuning in to our bodies gives us the opportunity to realize our dreams.

We long to travel in space. That desire stands at the heart of so much contemporary creative work. *Star Wars* and *Star Trek* sell out theaters and have spawned many multimillion dollar businesses. We seem to forget that we live on the most amazing, self-sustaining spaceship we have ever found in our universe. Every 24 hours we get a complete, panoramic view of the known universe. Every 365 days we travel around our sun on a virtual paradise that not only meets our essential needs for air, water, and food, but provides amenities such as hot and cold running water, heat and light at the flick of a switch, a cornucopia of amusements, and rapid travel all over the globe.

We move around our spaceship in amazing bodies, largely self-healing and self-sustaining given breathable air, drinkable water, and food. These bodies also form an ecosystem, a microuniverse that provides us with the ability to adapt to an almost infinite variety of variables.

Yet, we still find some room for complaint.

We want an ordered world in which we can predict the future, avoid surprises, and not have to work too hard. For centuries, science has endeavored to give us such a world.

Four hundred years ago Isaac Newton gave us a formula that worked marvelously. His theory of gravity and his laws of motion condensed into a formula: Force equals mass times acceleration ($F = ma$). This formula predicted movement of the planets and led the way to developing machines that did amazing things with much less human effort. When those theories made their way into medicine, we began describing the body as a machine that needed regular upkeep and occasional replacement of parts. Our ability to do these things has evolved exponentially over the last few decades. What we can do today to save and prolong lives was unimaginable a century ago.

A hundred years ago, Einstein came along and kicked the can of physics down the road to a place where prediction and technology became much more complex. Newton gave us predictability with one kind of energy, Force. Einstein explained that Energy (invisible) and mass (matter with substance) were equivalent at the speed of light squared ($E = mc^2$). Not only does that make our smart phones and magnetic resonance imaging equipment work, it also opened the door to chaos (mathematics) and unpredictable vagaries of the universe, such as intuition. We also learned that Force won't always work, and Energy harnessed from splitting atoms or from burning fossil fuels comes with a huge price in terms of the destruction of life as we know it.

Einstein believed that "God does not play dice with the universe," and he thought that quantum mechanics and relativity would still make prediction possible. Stephen Hawking, a few more theories and proofs farther down the road, said, "All the evidence points to [God] being an inveterate gambler, who throws the dice on every possible occasion" (Hawking, 1999). Indeed, given the properties of Hawking's specialty, black holes, "[God] sometimes confuses us by throwing [the dice] where they can't be seen" (Hawking, 1999). We humans still don't know everything, and, "God still has a few tricks up his sleeve" (Hawking, 1999).

Rather than taking this as bad news about the capriciousness of the universe, I choose instead to see it as a chance to get in the game. If you've read this far, you do know how I feel about play, especially with others! The question then becomes how we stay healthy and happy in this game of life.

I've often played quite hard—setting goals and jumping into new adventures. I find that doing so always enriches my life with lessons learned. In balance, I could say my life has been blessed with much joy. Many people have scoffed at such a positive attitude by bringing up examples of lives fraught with hardship and pain. I have had some of those moments, too.

In my fifties, I left behind my home of 25 years. In spite of the fact that I had moved closer to family and entered a legendary city full of unlimited opportunities, I found myself depressed, with all-too-frequent thoughts of suicide. I managed to stay in the game by staying connected to friends, family, and belief in a conscious universe. That universe put two books into my hands, and, serendipitously, I read them back to back. In *Deep Survival: Who Lives, Who Dies, and Why*, Laurence Gonzales recounts the stories of people who have survived against all odds, starting with his father, a pilot who was shot down behind enemy lines during World War II. From these stories he distills some rules for surviving adventure.

In *How We Choose to Be Happy: The 9 Choices of Extremely Happy People—Their Secrets, Their Stories*, Rick Foster and Greg Hicks travel around the world interviewing people described by friends, family, and neighbors as the "happiest people they know." From these interviews they come up with nine choices everyone makes in order to turn adversity or trauma into happiness.

The choices Gonzales ascribes to survivors and the ones Foster and Hicks discern for choosing happiness seem remarkably similar. Table 7.1 shows the two sets of choices they have identified for survival and happiness. Sustainable health requires both approaches. Making these kinds of choices every day pulls us out of feeling victimized by a health care system that all too often doesn't seem to care. We begin to tune into our own bodies, minds, and spirits. As soon as we choose happiness, we choose to live our lives more fully.

Table 7.1: Choosing Survival and Happiness

Survival choice	Happiness choice	Description
Perceive, believe	Intention	*Notice the funny and beautiful details. Go within to find opportunity.* Choose happiness over unhappiness.
Stay calm	Accountability	*Make use of fear, get angry, and keep a sense of humor.* Take control of your life.
Believe in success. Think, analyze, plan.	Identification	*Determine to do your best. Act with discipline and the expectation of success.* Identify which choices will make you happy.
Take correct decisive action	Centrality	*Take risks. Set attainable goals. Leave everything else behind.* Do what makes you happy, now.
Celebrate your successes.	Recasting	*Take great joy in the smallest success.* Find meaning in trauma and use it for energy.
See the beauty	Appreciation	*Appreciation relieves stress and provides information.* Transform the ordinary into something wonderful.
Count your blessings	Options	*Help others, even imaginary ones.* Be flexible enough to jump into the unknown.
Play	Giving	*Engage in the crisis as a game. Sing, count, recite, do math.* Do not expect a "return on investments."
Surrender	Truthfulness	*Accept pain and death.* Let go of external expectations and tune in to your own needs.
Do whatever is necessary. Never give up.	Synergy	*Use willpower and skills. Keep spirit alive with memory. Feel grateful for the experience.* Intention forms the center and keeps the other eight choices in balance.

We could think of these as rules for staying in the game when the dice don't roll our way. Luck changes all the time, and our ability to use powers of prediction to rig the game still eludes us.

On any adventure as precarious and unpredictable as life, it helps to have a compass. This book has endeavored to provide one. Our bodies can become our compass. When we care for and use our bodies as a compass we improve our odds for health and happiness.

This chapter offers one more practice, to lovingly cherish and polish our bodies, our personal compass. Figure 7.1 gives a general idea of how each element from the compass presents itself on our body, based loosely on the meridians of TCM. By using our hands, we can love ourselves up and keep track of the state of our own energetic vibrations for health and happiness. We follow the sequence in Figure 7.2 to move our hands over every part of our body.

We spend our entire journey through this lifetime in a body we received at birth. Most of us have spent plenty of time criticizing our bodies' perceived shortcomings—thighs, tummy, skin, hair, eyes, ears, and genes. We spend small fortunes trying to remedy these perceived flaws, and we berate ourselves when we cannot afford, complete, or persevere with a remedial regimen.

We can perceive our body as something flawed that needs fixing or as a constantly evolving and changing ecosystem that reflects our inner thoughts and emotions, as well as the conscious universe where we live and breathe. The former leads to discontent, whereas the latter can lead to wonder and joy. We can perceive each response of our body to the environment as a curious reaction to disease pathogens, toxins, and overuse. Each ache, pain, itch, extra pound, and sniffle heralds the many ways our body, as a microcosm of the universe, stands up to communicate and care for us.

Exercise 7.1: The Body Scan as Our Daily Conversation with the Conscious Universe

A daily body scan, done during bathing, toweling off, or putting on lotion, allows us to tune in to ancient wisdom, three million years of genetic adaptation alive in our bodies. It gives us a chance to interact lovingly with our bodies and sets us on a path of communication and cooperation, where our internal harmony synchronizes with external realities.

Each direction, each elemental energy of the Healing Compass, has a frequency relationship with specific body tissues and internal organs. As we run our hands over every part of our body, we become familiar with its changing responses. More sensitive than any piece of technology, our hands bring awareness of these changes and allow us to respond in ways that will support our health and well-being. Exploring the deeper meaning of these changes allows us to adjust our habits so that we can achieve vitality and happiness. We can assist our body's constant mission to repair and heal itself. All cells in our bodies, except for some neurons in our brains, replace themselves so that every 7 years or so we have what amounts to a completely new body.

Our hands can exquisitely sense changes, and they also have the power to heal. The centers of our palms resonate with Fire energy in many healing traditions, including our own. Presenting an open palm to a stranger indicates willingness to communicate. Pressing both palms together indicates respect. Look at the placement of hands in works of art. Hands communicate, and hands can heal. We can use ours to linger over problem areas with the intent to heal through love.

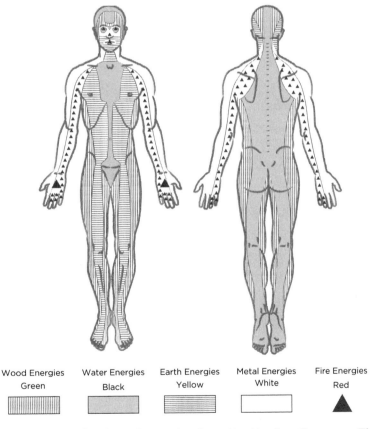

| Wood Energies | Water Energies | Earth Energies | Metal Energies | Fire Energies |
| Green | Black | Yellow | White | Red |

Figure 7.1 The body's reflection of energies from the Healing Compass. The patterns relate to the colors of elements in the Healing Compass Figure 1.1 and indicate which of the five elements resonates with that section of the body.

We can repeat this sequence as often as feels good. Each time, use a loving touch that covers every inch of skin.

1. Begin with our right hand over the heart. Connect to Fire energy. Fire energy from our right palm connects with Earth energy. Like lava, it rises up over the front of our left shoulder and flows down the inside of our arm, forearm, and hand, coalescing into rock over the left little, ring, and middle fingers.

2. Continuing with the right hand, draw Metal energy like stardust over the back of our left thumb and fingers, along the back of our hand, forearm, and triceps across our shoulder to the back of our neck.

3. Our left hand rises to meet the right hand and continues the flow of energy over our right shoulder. Imagine another stream of lava flowing down the inside of our right arm, coalescing into rock as it passes the little, ring, and middle fingers.

4. With the left hand move stardust down the back of your right thumb, hand, forearm, and triceps, to the back of your right shoulder.

5. Bring our right hand to our left shoulder and use both hands to caress our ears. Our hands uncross over the top of our head, and move over our face, pulling Earth, Wood, Water, Metal, and Fire energies down the sides of our neck.

6. Each hand moves under its corresponding armpit and reaches to the top of our back, as far as we can reach.

7. Like a waterfall, our hands smooth down both sides of the back over the kidneys and buttocks, once again picking up Wood and Earth energies to become a primordial ooze giving birth to life as they travel down the outside of our thighs, legs and feet.

8. Move that oozing life energy to caress between each toe and imagine it traveling like a vine between the first and second toes, over the arches of our feet, along the inside of our legs and thighs, through our genital area to ground itself in the receptive Earth energy of our belly buttons.

This body scan lends itself very well to daily washing up and putting on moisturizer. We can use this sequence when we suds up and rinse off in the shower. Repeat it again when toweling dry, and again when putting on a moisturizing

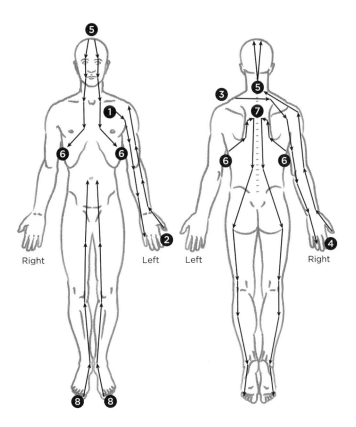

Figure 7.2 Sequence for the Body Scan
1. Right hand over heart. Rise over left shoulder and flow down the inside of arm, forearm, and hand, to left little, ring, and middle fingers.
2. Continue with right hand over the back of left thumb and fingers, along back of hand, forearm, triceps across shoulder to back of neck.
3. Left hand rises to meet right hand and continues the right shoulder, down the inside of right arm to little, ring, and middle fingers.
4. Left hands moves over back of right thumb, hand, forearm, and triceps, to back of right shoulder.
5. Right hand to left shoulder, both hands over ears, uncross over top of head, and move over face down the sides of neck.
6. Hands move under armpits and reach as far as possible up the back.
7. Hands move down both sides of the back over the kidneys and buttocks and travel down the back of our thighs, legs and feet.
8. Caress between each toe, over the arches of feet, along the inside of legs and thighs through genital area to belly button.

lotion. As part of a daily routine, the scan guides us into using our body to communicate with the universal elements of the Healing Compass.

It helps us become familiar with our own marvelous and constantly healing body. We can note its changes, lumps, and bumps as they appear and disappear. The location of these spots might give us some insight into suppressed emotions. We can be curious about unexplored grief when a bruise appears on the underside of our forearm, or wonder what's making us angry aside from that piece of furniture on which we just stubbed our toe. Take note of sore spots. Is fear of something raising its voice in our body? Pain, cold, and fear all resonate with Water energy. Give those spots extra love and warmth from the fiery palm of your hand.

If we have trouble bending over to touch our toes, we can do it more easily by raising our foot onto the side of the tub or a low chair. We can use this opportunity to gently stretch muscles and tendons. Reaching as high as we can on our back stretches more tendons. Go easy. This is a loving ritual, not a workout at the gym. Our flexibility returns as we do these simple, gentle stretches every day.

When we improve our odds for health and happiness, it turns out we also improve the health and happiness of those around us, including the environment of living and nonliving beings that makes our planet home.

Beliefs create thoughts.
Thoughts create emotions.
Emotions create actions.
Actions create health.

When we *believe* the universe revolves around us, we *think* our desires and actions will somehow enable us to control it. We get *angry* when things don't go our way and *regret* whatever decisions we made that somehow caused us to lose control. We *worry* endlessly over how to control the next event on our path to fame and fortune. We *fear* the unknown. We stress over micromanaging, lash out at people around us, use precious energy searching for the right words and deeds, and put off happiness and enjoyment until that perfect moment in the future when we have everything under control. These emotions and behaviors lead to many chronic illnesses.

When we *believe* ourselves part of an infinite network connected to a conscious universe, we can relinquish the driver's seat. We can *choose* to see the *beauty* around us, feel *gratitude* for every success and gift that comes our way, stop worrying, and have *faith* that each step we take will mean something. We will smile and laugh more often, attract a supportive group of friends and family, use our energy for healing, and enjoy each moment we can. These behaviors lead to health and happiness.

Belief in the body as a machine leads to thinking we can fix or replace just about anything. We get angry when that doesn't always work out, we worry about how to keep it all going as long as possible, and we fear that each ache and pain is the beginning of the end. We live lives as risk-free as possible and depend on a host of costly technicians and products to keep us going for as long as possible. Our taxes increase to cover the costs associated with the high-tech prices of modern life, including our health care, and we still die.

Belief in the body as an ecosystem leads to curiosity about just who is in here with us. We take joy in learning to make friends with this body, to play with it and find out what we can do together. We take some risks and provide tender loving care to the inevitable scrapes and bruises we'll sustain along the way. We can accept help from others when it feels right for our body, out of an internal sense of peace, rather than externally driven fears. We still pay taxes and die, but we lose our sense of desperation that we have to maintain hugely high-tech industries just to get by.

Our environment benefits from our ability to sustain our own health. When we watch the wind blow we learn to love and protect wild places more than the technology that often depends on destroying them.

When we turn off our gadgets to get a good night's sleep we heal faster, have more energy, and come up with creative solutions to environmental problems that impact our health and the health of our fellow travelers on this planet.

When we begin eating foods we love, we find that taste matters. When we know the origins of our food, we make healthier choices, both for ourselves and for the environment. Chemical pesticides and fertilizers just taste nasty! No processed sweetener will ever match the flavor of ripe fruit we pick right off the tree.

Eliminating what we don't need and want from our homes makes us more parsimonious consumers and more conscious contributors to our growing landfills.

Kindling the hearth of love and friendship warms our hearts and those of the people we love.

We all travel our life's journey one small step or decision at a time. People who have survived life-threatening or traumatic experiences and people who have reached the pinnacle of success did so by making one choice after another. Survival and happiness come to us when we choose life and healing, and then take the next logical or intuitive step.

Choose to feel joy at the miracle of life itself. Take pleasure in the only body we will get for this lifetime. Love it up!

Exercise 7.2: Doing the Body Scan with Our Children

Touch nourishes children. We know that without frequent physical contact infants do not thrive. (Ardiel, Rankin, 2010). Severe lack of physical contact, sustained in orphanages, has shown to lower intelligence, cause mental illness and potentially even result in death (The St. Petersburg—USA Orphanage Research Team, 2008)

As parents and caregivers we need to touch our children in loving ways. We can wash, dry, and put lotion on a child in the same way we would do for our self. Bathing and caressing our children also gives us a chance to examine their skin for rashes, bruises, or cuts.

Rashes may indicate that a child has sensitivity or allergies to foods or other elements in the environment. As children begin walking, running, and climbing, they are sure to get bruises and cuts on knees, elbows, foreheads, and chins. When we find cuts and bruises in places unlikely to result from a typical fall, question how these might have occurred and seek help from a health care provider in treating any rashes, cuts, and bruises that do not heal quickly or seem unusual in origin.

Pay attention to different feelings that come up when we caress our child or our self. If doing so makes us uncomfortable, we might consider visiting a therapist to try to address these feelings and become more comfortable with our own body so that we can care for our children in more loving ways.

Many places offer baby massage courses. These courses can help us feel more confident when touching our child in loving ways. As they get older children can learn to do the body scan for themselves.

Exercise 7.3: Doing the Body Scan with Elders

Touch remains important to our ability to thrive and stay healthy throughout life. Elders often suffer from lack of touch. Friends die and family moves away. As our ability to care for ourselves diminishes we sometimes find ourselves at the mercy of caregivers who are overworked, underpaid, impatient, and in a hurry. For many elders, this is the only kind of touch they receive and in the absence of other, more loving, kinds of touch they may resist becoming more independent in self-care simply because they need some form of daily physical contact with other people.

Elders often appreciate having someone smoothly caress their arms and hands. We can use the pattern of the first part of the body scan to do this. We can do it through clothing without overreaching any intimacy boundaries.

If we care for an elder by helping them wash up we can follow these same patterns to balance and smooth out their energy with washcloths, towels, and lotion. Pay attention to lumps, bumps, and sore spots.

Skin gets thin and fragile as we age, so elders may suffer cuts and bruises with minimal contact. Most often these occur as they bump into furniture or walls. Ask them about any suspicious bruising or cuts. Sometimes they forget to mention falls or other mishaps until asked. The incident that caused the injury may have gone unnoticed or receded from memory.

We can extend our loving energy to elders. As they are, so we may be. Touch them as we would wish to be touched.

Appendix A:
Sugar by Many Other Names

Sugars are carbohydrates made up of one or more molecules. Glucose, fructose, and galactose are single-molecule sugars (monosaccharides) that occur naturally or through manufacturing processes. Sucrose, lactose, and maltose are double-molecule sugars (disaccharides) made up of various combinations of glucose, fructose, and galactose, and they also occur naturally or through manufacturing processes. Starches consist of multiple sugar molecules (polysaccharides) that allow plants to store excess sugar. Normal digestion and manufacturing processes break these starches into simpler forms of sugar.

Our bodies require glucose as fuel. All cells in our body can metabolize this sugar into energy. Ribose and deoxyribose are sugars that make up our RNA and DNA. Our bodies process and recombine the foods we eat to make these essential sugars. The following list defines many common foods and food additives containing sugar.

COMMON NAME	GLUCOSE	FRUCTOSE	GALACTOSE	DESCRIPTION
Agave nectar or syrup	Some	Mostly		Commercially produced from several species of agave plants. Sweeter than honey and thinner in consistency. Exact percentages of fructose and glucose vary from vendor to vendor.
Brown rice syrup	100%			Made by fermenting cooked rice with enzymes (usually from dried barley sprouts) to break down the starches, then strained and reduced by cooking to reach desired consistency. Contains 52% maltotriose (a trisaccharide made up of three glucose molecules).

COMMON NAME	GLUCOSE	FRUCTOSE	GALACTOSE	DESCRIPTION
Brown sugar	46–48%	46–48%		Sugar crystals contained in molasses syrup with natural flavor and color made from sugar cane. Some refiners make brown sugar by adding syrup to refined white sugar.
Cane sugar, cane crystals, and evaporated cane juice	50%	50%		Comes from the processing of sugar cane into table sugar.
Coconut or palm sugar	~50%	~50%		Made from coconut palm flowers. Has some trace amounts of minerals.
Confectioner's sugar, or powdered sugar	50%	50%		Finely ground sucrose crystals mixed with a small amount of cornstarch.
Corn syrups, corn sweeteners, and crystalline fructose	2–58%	42–98%		Produced by the action of enzymes and/or acids on cornstarch, splitting that starch into sugar components. Also contain dextrose, water, and trace minerals.
Dextrose	100%			A form of glucose, commercially made from corn starch by the action of heat and acids, or enzymes. Blended with regular sugar and many powdered artificial sweeteners.
FRUCTOSE		100%		A single sugar molecule found naturally in honey and fruits. Sweeter than sucrose. Fructose requires the liver to metabolize it into usable energy for the body. A synthesized version, refined by the food industry decades ago, created a product known as high fructose corn syrup.
Fruit juice concentrates		Mostly		Made from dehydrating fruit juices and using them as sweeteners.
GALACTOSE			100%	A single-molecule sugar that occurs naturally in the body. Combines with glucose to form lactose, the sugar found in milk.
GLUCOSE	100%			A single-molecule sugar occurring naturally in all living organisms and used for energy. Manufacturers create glucose by processing starches from a wide variety of plants including corn, maize, rice, wheat, cassava, corn husk and sago.

COMMON NAME	GLUCOSE	FRUCTOSE	GALACTOSE	DESCRIPTION
High-fructose corn syrup (HFCS)	42–50%	50–55%		A sweetener made from cornstarch. The amounts of fructose vary with the manufacturer. An enzyme-linked process increases the fructose content, thus making HFCS sweeter than regular corn syrup.
Honey	Varies	Varies		An invert sugar formed by bees' enzymes from gathered nectar. Honey contains fructose, glucose, maltose, and sucrose.
Invert sugar	~50%	~50%		A mixture of glucose and fructose. Formed by splitting sucrose in a process called inversion. Prevents crystallization of cane sugar in candy making.
LACTOSE or milk sugar	Varies		Varies	A double-molecule sugar consisting of glucose and galactose. Occurs naturally in the milk of mammals. Manufactured from whey and skim milk for commercial purposes, primarily in the pharmaceutical industry.
MALTOSE	100%			A double-molecule sugar consisting of two glucose molecules. Made by fermenting barley grains and caramelizing them by heating sugar until it turns brown. The body breaks maltose into glucose very easily and rapidly.
Malt syrup	100%			Made from sprouting, fermenting, and caramelizing grains such as barley, and wheat. Also contains a little protein.
Maple syrup and sugar	50%	50%		Made by boiling the sap of sugar maple trees.
Molasses and blackstrap molasses	~50%	~50%		Produced as a by-product of processing sugar cane. Quality depends on the maturity of the sugar cane, the amount of sugar extracted, and the method of extraction. Blackstrap molasses contains the least amount of sugar as well as trace amounts of vitamins and significant amounts of calcium, magnesium, potassium, and iron; one tablespoon provides up to 20% of the daily value of each of those nutrients.

COMMON NAME	GLUCOSE	FRUCTOSE	GALACTOSE	DESCRIPTION
Muscovado and panela	~50%	~50%		Whole cane sugar extracted by mechanical processes, heated, and cooled, forming small brown grainy crystals of pure dried sugar cane juice that retain their molasses content.
Raw sugar	~50%	~50%		Coarse, granulated crystals of sucrose formed from the evaporation of sugar cane juice. True raw sugar contains impurities and cannot be sold in grocery stores due to FDA regulations.
Sweet sorghum syrup or sorghum molasses	~50%	~50%		Made from sorghum (in the same grass family as sugar cane) in much the same way molasses is made from sugar cane and sugar beets.
Sucanat and Rapadura	~50%	~50%		Brand names for a variety of whole cane sugar extracted by mechanical processes. Similar to panela and muscovado, it retains its molasses content.
SUCROSE or table sugar	49.9%	49.9%		Made from sugar cane or sugar beets.
Turbinado sugar	~50%	~50%		Raw sugar made by spinning in a cylinder or turbine. Brown but paler than brown sugar with a subtle molasses flavor.

Appendix B:
Sugar Substitutes

Sugar substitutes, also called artificial sweeteners, take the place of sucrose (table sugar) and other sugars (see Appendix A) to sweeten foods and beverages. The U.S. Food and Drug Administration (FDA) regulates artificial sweeteners through the Food Additives Amendment to the Food, Drug, and Cosmetic Act, passed by Congress in 1958. This law requires the FDA to approve food additives, including artificial sweeteners, before they can be made available for sale in the United States.

Studies show conflicting evidence of potential harm caused by sugar substitutes. Most have few or no calories, so contribute nothing in terms of nutritional value to our foods. Many are made from ingredients we would never consider eating under normal circumstances. Recent studies indicate that despite their lack of calories, most sugar substitutes seem to contribute to weight gain rather than prevent it (Azad et al., 2017). Sugar substitutes do not seem to contribute to tooth decay as sugars do.

The following list gives the names and some information about common sugar substitutes.

CHEMICAL NAME	TRADE NAMES	SWEETNESS INDEX (COMPARED TO SUGAR)	COOKING OR BAKING	COMMONLY FOUND IN	DESCRIPTION
Acesulfame K	Sunett and Sweet One	200	Yes	Foods and beverages (protein shakes). Pharmaceutical products (chewable and liquid medications)	Accidentally discovered by a chemist in 1967. Has a slightly bitter aftertaste, especially at high concentrations. Blended with other sweeteners (usually sucralose or aspartame) to give a more sugar-like taste. Each sweetener masks the other's aftertaste.
Aspartame	NutraSweet, AminoSweet, Equal, and Candarel	180	No	Approximately 6000 consumer foods and beverages, diet sodas and other soft drinks, instant breakfasts, breath mints, cereals, sugar-free chewing gum, cocoa mixes, frozen desserts, gelatin desserts, juices, laxatives, chewable vitamins supplements, milk drinks, pharmaceutical drugs and supplements, shake mixes, tabletop sweeteners, teas, instant coffees, topping mixes, wine coolers, and yogurt.	First synthesized by a chemist in the course of producing an antiulcer drug in 1965. When eaten, aspartame breaks down into natural residual components, including aspartic acid, phenylalanine, methanol, and further breakdown products including formaldehyde and formic acid. Must be avoided by people with the genetic condition PKU.

CHEMICAL NAME	TRADE NAMES	SWEETNESS INDEX (COMPARED TO SUGAR)	COOKING OR BAKING	COMMONLY FOUND IN	DESCRIPTION
Cyclamate	Sweet'N Low and Sugar Twin (outside U.S.A.)	40	Yes		Banned by the FDA for use in the United States, but used as an approved sweetener in over 55 countries including Canada. Discovered in 1937 by graduate student working in the lab on the synthesis of anti-fever medication. Often combined with other artificial sweeteners, especially saccharin to mask the off-tastes of both sweeteners.
Maltitol	Maltisorb, Maltisweet and Lesys	0.9	Yes	Sugarless hard candies, chewing gum, chocolate candies, baked goods and ice cream. Often replaces fat due to creamy texture.	A sugar alcohol or polyol, made from maltose. Used to replace table sugar because it has fewer calories, does not promote tooth decay, and has a somewhat lesser effect on blood glucose. Like other sugar alcohols, large quantities can have a laxative effect.
Lo Han Guo	Sweet Sensation, Nectresse, Lakanto	300	Yes	Still new in U.S. manufacturing	Extracted from monk fruits. Used in China for 800 years as sweetener and herbal medicine. Often bulked up with other sweeteners.

CHEMICAL NAME	TRADE NAMES	SWEETNESS INDEX (COMPARED TO SUGAR)	COOKING OR BAKING	COMMONLY FOUND IN	DESCRIPTION
Mannitol		0.5	Yes	Food and pharmaceuticals. Keeps products moisture-free.	A sugar alcohol or polyol, can act as diuretic agent and weak renal vasodilator. Originally isolated from the secretions of the flowering ash tree. Synthesized through the hydrogenation of fructose, or extracted from a wide variety of plants.
Neotame	Newtame	8000	Yes	Diet soft drinks and low-calorie foods	Produced by the NutraSweet Company. A recent addition to FDA's list of approved artificial sweeteners. Developed specifically as an artificial sweetener. Lowers the cost of production because lower quantities achieve the same sweetening. Body appears to rapidly metabolize, completely eliminate and not accumulate this sweetener.
Saccharin	Sweet'N Low (in U.S.A.)	300	Yes	Beverages, candies, biscuits, medicines, and toothpaste	Discovered by a chemist working on coal tar derivatives in 1878. Commercialized not long after its discovery. Sugar shortages during World War I led to widespread use. Popularity increased during the 1960s and 1970s. Has a bitter or metallic aftertaste at high concentrations.

CHEMICAL NAME	TRADE NAMES	SWEETNESS INDEX (COMPARED TO SUGAR)	COOKING OR BAKING	COMMONLY FOUND IN	DESCRIPTION
Sorbitol	Glucitol, Isomalt, lycasin, Sorbogem and Sorbo	0.55	Yes	Candies, baked goods, and chocolates	A sugar alcohol or polyol metabolized slowly by the body. Obtained by reduction of glucose found in apples, pears, peaches, and prunes.
Stevia	Truvia, PureVia, Steviva, SweetLeaf	300	Yes	Teas, candies, chewing gum, soft drinks, flavored waters, and soy sauce	Stevia rebaudiana, grows in subtropical and tropical regions of North and South America. Used by native healers to treat diabetes. Bitter or licorice-like aftertaste diminishes with low concentrations of extracts. Ground into a green powder or processed as white powder or liquid.
Sucralose	Splenda, Sukrana, SucraPlus, Candys, Cukren and Nevella	600	Yes	Over 4000 low-fat products, including cereals and cereal bars; puddings, ice cream, popsicles; canned fruit, reduced-calorie baked goods, candy; juice, iced and hot tea, diet soda, coffee beverages; flavored milk, yogurt, coffee creamer; syrups, jams, jellies, and condiments; nutritional products and dietary supplements.	Discovered in 1976 researching ways to use sucrose in insecticides. Does not break it down and body excretes it whole. No nutritive (or caloric) value. Does not break down in environment, currently found in wastewater.

CHEMICAL NAME	TRADE NAMES	SWEETNESS INDEX (COMPARED TO SUGAR)	COOKING OR BAKING	COMMONLY FOUND IN	DESCRIPTION
Xylitol	Polysweet Xylosweet	1	Yes	Chewing gum, peanut butter, breath mints, mouthwash, candies, toothpaste, tooth whiteners, chewable vitamins.	Naturally occurring sugar alcohol sweetener made from hardwood or maize or extracted from various berries, oats, and mushrooms, corn husks and sugar cane husks also used to make biofuels. Temporary gastrointestinal side effects, such as bloating, flatulence, and diarrhea, diminish with frequent consumption. Toxic to dogs.

References

Alexander, B. K. (2011). *The Globalization of Addiction: A Study in Poverty of the Spirit.* New York: Oxford University Press.

American Occupational Therapy Association. (2017). Occupational Therapy Practice Framework: Domain and Process, 3rd ed. *American Journal of Occupational Therapy, 62*(6), 625–688.

Anderson, L. (2015, April 28). *6 words that will end picky eating.* Retrieved February 23, 2018, from Huffington Post: https://wwww.huffingtonpost.com/the-mid/6-words-that-will-end-picky-eating_b_7139710.html

Azad, M. B., Abou-Setta, A. M., Chauhan, B. F., Rabbani, R., Lys, J., Copstein, L., et al. (2017, July 17). Nonnutritive sweeteners and cardiometabolic health: A systematic review and meta-analysis of randomized controlled trials and prospective cohort studies. *CMAJ, 189*(28), E929–E939.

Ardiel, E.L., Rankin, C.H. (2010) The importance of touch in development. *Paediatr Child Health, 15*(3):153-156.

Bernstein, R. K. (2011). *Dr. Bernstein's Diabetes Solution: The Complete Guide to Achieving Normal Blood Sugars* (Kindle ed.). New York: Little, Brown.

Breuning, L. G. (2017). *The Science of Positivity: Stop Negative Thought Patterns by Changing Your Brain Chemistry* (Kindle ed.). Avon, MA: Adams Media.

Brogan, K. (2016). *A Mind of Your Own: The Truth About Depression and How Women Can Heal Their Bodies to Reclaim Their Lives* (Kindle ed.). New York: Harper Wave.

Burghardt, G. M. (2015). Play in fishes, frogs, and reptiles. *Current Biology, 25*(1), R9–R10.

Burr, C. (2003). *The Emperor of Scent: A True Story of Perfume and Obsession.* New York: Random House.

Carlson, J. B. (1975). *Lodestone compass: Chinese or Olmec primacy.* Retrieved December 23, 2017, from jstor.org: http://www.jstor.org/stable/1740186?origin=JSTOR-pdf&seq=1#page_scan_tab_contents

Cartwright, R. (2010). *The Twenty-Four Hour Mind: The Role of Sleep and Dreaming in Our Emotional lives.* New York: Oxford University Press.

Centers for Disease Control. (2017, April). *Long-term trends in diabetes.* Retrieved December 23, 2017, from cdc.gov: https://www.cdc.gov/diabetes/statistics/slides/long_term_trends.pdf

Centers for Medicare and Medicaid Services. (2016). *NHE fact sheet.* Retrieved December 23, 2017, from CMS.gov: https://www.cms.gov/research-statistics-data-and-systems/statistics-trends-and-reports/nationalhealthexpenddata/nhe-fact-sheet.html

Chida, Y., Sudo, N., & Kubo, C. (2006, Jan 21). *Does stress exacerbate liver disease?*

Retrieved Dec 26, 2017, from National Center for Biotechnology Information: https://www.ncbi.nlm.nih.gov/pubmed/16460474

Cilley, M. (2002). *Sink Reflections.* New York: Bantam Books.

Claus, S. P., Guillou, H., & Ellero-Simatos, S. (2016, May 4). *The gut microbiota: A major player in the toxicity of environmental pollutants.* Retrieved Nov 25, 2017, from Nature: https://www.nature.com/articles/npjbiofilms20163

Cline, E. H. (2014). *1177 B.C.: The Year Civilization Collapsed.* Princeton, NJ: Princeton University Press.

Cohen, S., Conduit, R., Lockley, S. W., Rajaratnam, S. M., & Cornish, K. M. (2014). The relationship between sleep and behavior in autism spectrum disorder (ASD): A review. *Journal of Neurodevelopmental Disorders, 6*(44), 1866–1955.

Craig, J. M., Logan , A. C., & Prescott, S. L. (2016, January 13). *Natural environments, nature relatedness and the ecological theater: Connecting satellites and sequencing to shinrin-yoku.* Retrieved December 25, 2017, from Journal of Physiological Anthropology: https://jphysiolanthropol.biomedcentral.com/articles/10.1186/s40101-016-0083-9

Crawford, M. (2009). *Shop Class as Soul Craft: An Inquiry into the Value of Work.* New York: Penguin Press.

Cytowick, R. E. (2015, June 9). *Your brain on screens.* Retrieved February 8, 2018, from The American Interest: https://www.the-american-interest.com/2015/06/09/your-brain-on-screens/

Doelling, K. B., & Poeppel, D. (2015, Oct 26). *Cortical entrainment to music and its modulation by expertise.* Retrieved Dec 26, 2017, from PNAS Plus: Biological Sciences: Neuroscience: http://www.pnas.org/content/112/45/E6233.abstract

Eisenstein, C. (2011). *Sacred Economics: Money, Gift, and Society in the Age of Transition* (Kindle ed.). Berkley, CA: Evolver Editions.

Eisenstein, C. (2013). *Ascent of Humanity: Civilization and the Human Sense of Self.* Berkeley, CA: North Atlantic Books.

Emory, N. J., & Clayton, N. S. (2015, January 5). Do birds have the capacity for fun? *Current Biology, 25*(1), R16–R20.

Ezard, J. (2000, October 24). *The story of Dr Jekyll, Mr Hyde and Fanny, the angry wife who burned the first draft.* Retrieved February 11, 2018, from The Guardian: https://www.theguardian.com/uk/2000/oct/25/books.booksnews

Forrestal, L. J. (2009, Feb 23). *The rise and fall of Crisco.* Retrieved Dec 27, 2017, from WestonAPrice.org: https://www.westonaprice.org/health-topics/modern-foods/the-rise-and-fall-of-crisco/

Foster, R., & Hicks, G. (1999). *How We Choose to Be Happy: The 9 Choices of Extremely Happy People—Their Secrets, Their Stories.* New York: Perigee Books.

Franquemont, A. (2009). *Respect the Spindle: Spin Infinite Yarns with One Amazing Tool.* Loveland, CO: Interweave Press.

Gleason, J. (1992). *Oya: In Praise of an African Goddess.* New York: Harper Collins.

Goleman, D., & Davidson, R. (2017). *Altered Traits: Science Reveals How Meditation Changes Your Mind, Brain, and Body* (Kindle ed.). New York: Random House.

Gonzales, L. (2005). *Deep Survival: Who Lives, Who Dies, and Why.* New York: W. W. Norton.

Gowlett, J. A. (2016, Jan 18). *The discovery of fire by humans: A long and convoluted process.* Retrieved Nov 3, 2017, from Royal Society Publishing: http://rstb.royalsocietypublishing.org/content/371/1696/20150164

Gray, P. (2013). *Free to Learn: Why Unleashing the Instinct to Play Will Make Our Children Happier, More Self-Reliant, and Better Students for Life* (Kindle ed.). New York: Basic Books.

Greene, D. P., & Roberts, S. L. (2017). *Kinesiology: Movement in the Context of Activity* (3rd ed.). St. Louis, MO: Elsevier.

Greer, J. M. (2016). *Retrotopia* (Kindle ed.). Danville, IL: Founder's House.

Guimarães, A. P. (2004, January). *Mexico and the early history of magnetism.* Retrieved December 24, 2017, from ResearchGate: https://www.researchgate.net/publication/26475637_Mexico_and_the_early_history_of_magnetism

Gunders, D. (2017, August 16). *Wasted: How America is losing up to 40 percent of its food from farm to fork to landfill.* Retrieved February 16, 2018, from National Resources Defense Council: https://www.nrdc.org/resources/wasted-how-america-losing-40-percent-its-food-farm-fork-landfill

Hallberg, L., Bjorn-Rasmussen, E., Rossander, L., & Suwanik, R. (1977, Apr 30). *Iron absorption from southeast Asian diets.* Retrieved Aug 23, 2017, from PubMed.gov: https://www.ncbi.nlm.nih.gov/pubmed/851082

Hamley, S. (2014, November 30). *Did hunter-gatherers eat at least 100g of fibre per day?* Retrieved February 15, 2018, from Stephen Hamley: http://www.stevenhamley.com.au/2014/11/did-hunter-gatherers-eat-at-least-100g.html

Hawking, S. (1999). *Does God play dice?* Retrieved Dec 19, 2017, from Hawking.org: http://www.hawking.org.uk/does-god-play-dice.html

Hoge, E. A., Chen, M. M., Orr, E., Metcalf, C. A., Fischer, L. E., Pollack, M. H., et al. (2013, August). Loving-Kindness Meditation practice associated with longer telomeres in women. *Brain, Behavior, and Immunity, 32*, 159–163.

Hume, L. (2004, March). Accessing the eternal: Dreaming "the dreaming" and ceremonial performance. *Zygon, 39*(1), 237–258.

Hutchinson, L. (2013, July 26). *The Rolling Stones' "(I Can't Get No) Satisfaction."* Retrieved February 11, 2018, from Performing Songwriter: http://performingsongwriter.com/rolling-stones-satisfaction/

Hyman, M. (2006). *Ultrametabolism.* New York: Atria Books.

Hyman, M. (2016). *Eat Fat, Get Thin: Why the Fat We Eat is the Key to Sustained Weight Loss and Vibrant Health* (Kindle ed.). New York: Little, Brown.

Jaffe, E. (2006, December) *Old World, High Tech.* Retrieved from Smithsonian Magazine: https://www.smithsonianmag.com/science-nature/old-world-high-tech-141284744/

Kanterman, T., Juda, M., Merrow, M., & Roenneburg, T. (2007, Nov 20). *The human circadian clock's seasonal adjustment is disrupted by daylight saving time.* Retrieved Nov 6, 2017, from Current Biology: http://www.cell.com/current-biology/abstract/S0960-9822%2807%2902086-6

Kaplan, M. (1976, July 19). Dalai Lama's brother, now a Jerseyan, enjoys his job as a school janitor. *New York Times*, p. 46.

Katz, S. E. (2003). *Wild Fermentation: The Flavor, Nutrition, and Craft of Live-Culture Foods.* White River Junction, VT: Chelsea Green Publishing.

Katzen, M., & Edelson, M. (2015). *The Healthy Mind Cookbook: Big-Flavor Recipes to Enhance Brain Function, Mood, Memory, and Mental Clarity.* Berkeley, CA: Ten Speed Press.

Kayser, M. S., & Biron, D. (2016, May). Sleep and development in genetically tractable model organisms. *Genetics*, 21–33.

Keys, A. (1980). *Seven countries: A multivariate analysis of death and coronary heart disease.* Cambridge, MA: Harvard University Press.

Kimmerer, R. W. (2015). *Braiding Sweetgrass: Indigenous Wisdom, Scientific Knowledge and the Teachings of Plants* (Kindle ed.). Minneapolis, MN: Milkweed Editions.

Kingston, K. (1997). *Creating Sacred Space with Feng Shui: Learn the Art of Space Clearing and Bring New Energy into Your Life.* New York: Broadway Books.

Kleitman, N. (1952, November). Sleep. *Scientific American, 187*(5), 34–39.

Krisch, K. (2014, Jun 10). *Attention restoration theory & nature: Let's solve problems. . . .* Retrieved Dec 26, 2017, from Positiive Psychology Program: https://positivepsychologyprogram.com/attention-restoration-theory-nature-lets-solve-problems/

Kuntsler, J. H. (2009). *World Made by Hand: A Novel* (Kindle ed.). New York: Grove Press.

Lansing, A. (2014). *Endurance: Shackleton's Incredible Voyage.* New York: Basic Books.

Le Billon, Karen. (2012). *French Kids Eat Everything: How Our Family Moved to France, Cured Picky Eating, Banned Snacking, and Discovered 10 Simple Rules for Raising Happy, Healthy Eaters.* (Kindle ed.) New York: William Morrow.

Leidoff, J. (1977). *The Continuum Concept: In Search Of Happiness Lost* (Kindle ed.). Cambridge, MA: Perseus Books.

Levy, F. (2012, Jan 11). *Mirror neurons, birdsong, and human language: A hypothesis.* Retrieved Dec 6, 2017, from Frontiers in Psychiatry: https://www.frontiersin.org/articles/10.3389/fpsyt.2011.00078/full

Li, Q. (2009, March 25). *Effect of forest bathing on human immune function.* Retrieved December 26, 2017, from National Center for Biotechnology Information: https://www.ncbi.nlm.nih.gov/pmc/articles/PMC2793341/

Longo, V. (2018). *The Longevity Diet: Discover the New Science Behind Stem Cell Activation and Regeneration to Slow Aging, Fight Disease, and Optimize Weight* (Kindle ed.). New York: Avery.

Louv, R. (2008). *Last Child in the Woods: Saving Our Children from Nature Deficit Disorder.* New York: Workman.

Lu, N., & Schaplowsky, E. (2015). *Digesting the Universe: A Revolutionary Framework for Healthy Metabolism Function.* New York: Tao of Healing Publishing.

Ludwig, David S. (2007). *Ending the Food Fight: Guide Your Child to a Healthy Weight in a Fast Food/Fake Food World* (Kindle ed.). Boston: Houghton Mifflin.

Lustig, R. H. (2013). *Fat Chance: Beating the Odds Against Sugar, Processed Food, Obesity, and Disease* (Kindle ed.). New York: Hudson Street Press.

Maas, J. B., & Davis, H. (2013). *Sleep to Win: Secrets to Unlocking your Athletic Excellence in Every Sport.* Bloomington, IN: AuthorHouse.

Matthew, J. (2016, January 30). *Where do all the elements come from?* Retrieved May 16, 2018, from Futurism: https://futurism.com/where-do-all-the-elements-come-from/

McBride, N. C. (2008, May 4). *Cholesterol: Friend or foe?* Retrieved Dec 26, 2017, from WestonAPrice: https://www.westonaprice.org/health-topics/know-your-fats/cholesterol-friend-or-foe/#comments

McEwen, B. S. (2012). Stress and anxiety: Structural plasticity and epigenetic regulation as a consequence of stress. *Neuropharmacology, 62*(1), 3–12.

McEwen, B. S. (2008). Central effects of stress hormones in health and disease: understanding the protective and damaging effects of stress and stress mediators. *European Journal of Pharmacology.* 583(2-3): 174–185.

McGasko, J. (2014, January 23). *Her 'Midnight Pillow': Mary Shelley and the Creation of Frankenstein*. Retrieved February 11, 2019, from Biography: https://www.biography.com/news/mary-shelley-frankenstein-i-frankenstein-movie

Miller, A. (2005). *The Body Never Lies: The Lingering Effects of Hurtful Parenting* (Kindle ed.) (A. Jenkins, Trans.). New York: W. W. Norton.

Mirmiran, M., Scholtens, J., Van de Poll, N. E., Uylings, H. B., Van der Gugten, J., & Boer, G. J. (1983, April). Effects of experimental suppression of active (REM) sleep during early development upon adult brain and behavior in the rat. *Developmental Brain Research, 7*(2–3), 277–286.

Morisson, G. (2015, August 2). *The truth about Ultra HD 4K TV refresh rates*. Retrieved February 8, 2018, from C/Net: https://www.cnet.com/news/ultra-hd-4k-tv-refresh-rates/

National Center for Health Statistics. (2017, May). *Health, United States, 2016: With chartbook on long-term trends in health*. Retrieved December 23, 2017, from Centers for Disease Control: https://www.cdc.gov/nchs/data/hus/hus16.pdf#093

National Institute of Mental Health. (2016). *Any mental illness among U.S. adults*. Retrieved December 23, 2017, from nimh.nih.gov: https://www.nimh.nih.gov/health/statistics/prevalence/any-mental-illness-ami-among-us-adults.shtml

National Sleep Foundation. (n.d.). *Sleep hygiene*. Retrieved February 13, 2018, from National Sleep Foundation: https://sleepfoundation.org/sleep-topics/sleep-hygiene

Nestle, M., & Nesheim, M. (2012). *Why calories count: from science to politics* (Kindle ed.). Berkeley: University of California Press.

O'Grady, R. (2016). *150 Strong: A Pathway to a Different Future* (Kindle ed.). Beaufort, SC: Club Orlov Press.

Ody, P. (2017). *The Complete Medicinal Herbal*. New York: Skyhorse Publishing.

Olive, M. F., Koenig, H. N., Nannini, M. A., & Hodge, C. W. (2001, December 1). *Stimulation of endorphin neurotransmission in the nucleus accumbens by ethanol, cocaine, and amphetamine. J Neurosci. Dec 1;21(23):RC184*. Retrieved December 26, 2017, from The Journal of Neuroscience: http://www.jneurosci.org/content/21/23/RC184.long

Olkowicz, S., Kocourek, M., Radek , L., Porteš, M., Fitch, W., Herculano-Houzelc, S., et al. (2016, May 6). *Birds have primate-like numbers of neurons in the forebrain*. Retrieved Dec 6, 2017, from PNAS.org: http://www.pnas.org/content/113/26/7255

Organisation for Economic Co-Operation and Development. (2017). *Health spending 2016*. Retrieved December 23, 2017, from OECD.org: https://data.oecd.org/healthres/health-spending.htm

Organisation for Economic Co-Operation and Development. (2017). *Obesity update 2017*. Retrieved December 23, 2017, from OECD.org: https://www.oecd.org/els/health-systems/Obesity-Update-2017.pdf

Park, B. J., Kagawa, T., Kasetani, T., Tsunetsugu, Y., & Miyazaki, Y. (2009, May 2). *The physiological effects of Shinrin-yoku (taking in the forest or forest bathing): Evidence from field experiments in 24 forests across Japan*. Retrieved December 26, 2017, from National Center for Biotechnology Information: https://www.ncbi.nlm.nih.gov/pmc/articles/PMC2793346/

Polk, S. (2014, January 19). For the love of money. *New York Times Sunday Review*, p. SR1.

Pollan, M. (2013). *Cooked: A Natural History of Transformation* (Kindle ed.). New York: Penguin Press.

Popova, M. (n.d.). *How Mendeleev invented his periodic table in a dream*. Retrieved February 11, 2018, from Brain Pickings: https://www.brainpickings.org/2016/02/08/mendeleev-periodic-table-dream/

Porges, S. W. (2011). *The Polyvagal Theory: Neurophysiological Foundations of Emotions, Attachment, Communication, and Self-Regulation* (Kindle ed.). New York: W.W. Norton.

Prather, A. A., Hall, M., Fury, J. M., Ross, D. C., Muldoon, M. F., Cohen, S., et al. (2012, August 1). Sleep and antibody response to Hepatitis B vaccination. *Sleep, 35*(8), 1063–1069.

Prather, A. A., Janicki-Deverts, D., Hall, M. H., & Cohen, S. (2015, September 1). Behaviorally assessed sleep and susceptibility to the common cold. *Sleep, 38*(9), 1353–1359.

Price, W. A. (2008). *Nutrition and Physical Degeneration* (8th ed.). Lemon Grove, CA: Price-Pottenger Nutrition Foundation.

Robin, V., & Dominguez, J. (2018). *Your Money or Your Life: 9 Steps to Transforming Your Relationship with Money and Achieving Financial Independence* (rev. ed.). New York: Penguin Books.

Rosbash, M. (2003). A biological clock. *Daedalus, 132*(2), 27–36.

Rutherford, B. R. (2013). A randomized, prospective pilot study of patient expectancy and antidepressant outcome. *Psychological Medicine, 43*(5), 975–982.

Sahlins, M. (2017). *Stone Age Economics* (Kindle ed.). New York: Routledge.

Satter, E. (2008). *Secrets of Feeding a Healthy Family: How to Eat, How to Raise Good Eaters, How to Cook.* Madison, WI: Kelcy Press.

Satter, E. (2017). *Stop being hysterical about "obesity."* Retrieved December 2017, 2017, from ellynsatterinstitute.org: https://www.ellynsatterinstitute.org/family-meals-focus/11-update-stop-being-hysterical-about-obesity/

Schauss, M. (2015, June 30). *Toxicity and chronic illness.* Retrieved December 23, 2017, from westonaprice.org: https://www.westonaprice.org/health-topics/environmental-toxins/toxicity-and-chronic-illness/

Siegel, D. J. (2016). *Mind: A Journey into the Heart of Being Human* (Kindle ed.). New York: W. W. Norton.

Strickland, E., McCloskey, S., Ryberg, R. (2009). *Eating for Autism: The 10-Step Nutrition Plan to Help Treat Your Child's Autism, Asperger's or ADHD.* Boston: DaCapo Press.

Sundelin, T., Lekander, M., Sorjonen, K., & Axelsson, J. (2017, May 17). *Negative effects of restricted sleep on facial appearance and social appeal.* Retrieved February 9, 2009, from Royal Society Open Science: http://rsos.royalsocietypublishing.org/content/4/5/160918

Tara, S. (2017). *The Secret Life of Fat: The Science Behind the Body's Least Understood Organ* (Kindle Edition ed.). New York: W.W. Norton.

The St. Petersburg—USA Orphanage Research Team. (2008). The effects of early social-emotional and relationship experience on the development of young orphanage children. *Monographs of the Society for Research in Child Development, 73*(3), vii–295. http://doi.org/10.1111/j.1540-5834.2008.00483.x

Theofanopoulou, C., Boeckx, C., & Jarvis, E. (2017, Jul 20). *A hypothesis on a role of oxytocin in the social mechanisms of speech and vocal learning.* Retrieved Dec 5, 2017, from Royal Society Publishing.

Ulrich, R. S. (1984, Aprl 27). *View through a window may influence recovery from surgery.* Retrieved Dec 26, 2017, from Science Magazine: http://science.sciencemag.org/content/224/4647/420

U.S. Department of Health and Human Services, U.S. Department of Agriculture. (n.d.). *Dietary guidelines for Americans 2015–2020.* Retrieved February 15, 2018, from Health.gov: https://health.gov/dietaryguidelines/2015/guidelines/appendix-7/

Verghese, J., Lipton, R., Katz , M., Hall, C., Derby, C., Kuslansky, G., et al. (2003, Jun 19). *Leisure activities and the risk of dementia in the elderly.* Retrieved Dec 6, 2017, from NEJM.org: http://www.nejm.org/doi/full/10.1056/NEJMoa022252

Vincent, A. (2015, June 18). *Yesterday: The song that started as Scrambled Eggs.* Retrieved February 11, 2018, from The Telegraph: http://www.telegraph.co.uk/culture/music/the-beatles/11680415/Yesterday-the-song-that-started-as-Scrambled-Eggs.html

Viola, A. U., James, L. M., Schlangen, L. J., & Dijk, D.-J. (2008, August). Blue-enriched white light in the workplace improves self-reported alertness, performance and sleep quality. *Scandinavian Journal of Work, Environment & Health, 34*(4), 297–306.

Walker, M. (2017). *Why We Sleep: Unlocking the Power of Sleep and Dreams* (Kindle ed.). New York: Scribners.

Walsh, P. (2008). *Does This Clutter Make My Butt Look Fat? An Easy Plan for Losing Weight and Living More.* New York: Free Press.

White paper: Consequences of drowsy driving. (n.d.). Retrieved February 13, 2018, from National Sleep Foundation: https://sleepfoundation.org/white-paper-consequences-drowsy-driving

WHO Regional Office for Europe. (2016). *Urban green spaces and health.* Retrieved Dec 26, 2017, from World Health Organization Europe: http://www.euro.who.int/__data/assets/pdf_file/0005/321971/Urban-green-spaces-and-health-review-evidence.pdf?ua=1

Wise, J. (2009, March 18). *Danish night shift workers with breast cancer awarded compensation.* Retrieved February 9, 2018, from The BMJ: https://doi.org/10.1136/bmj.b1152

Wohlleben, P. (2016). *The Hidden Life of Trees: What They Feel, How They Communicate—Discoveries from a Secret World* (Kindle ed.) (J. Billinghurst, Trans.). Vancouver: Greystone Books.

Wolverton, B. C., Johnson, A., & Bounds, K. (1989, September 15). *Interior landscape plants for indoor air pollution abatement.* Retrieved December 26, 2017, from NASA Technical Reports Server: https://ntrs.nasa.gov/search.jsp?R=19930073077#

Yudkin, J., & Lustig, R. H. (2017). *Pure, White and Deadly: How Sugar is Killing Us and What We Can Do to Stop It* (International ed.). London, UK: Penguin.

Index

In this index, *f* denotes figure and *t* denotes table.